Putting a Name to It
Diagnosis in Contemporary Society

SECOND EDITION

Annemarie Goldstein Jutel

Johns Hopkins University Press
Baltimore

© 2011, 2024 Johns Hopkins University Press
All rights reserved. Published 2024
Printed in the United States of America on acid-free paper
9 8 7 6 5 4 3 2 1

Johns Hopkins University Press
2715 North Charles Street
Baltimore, Maryland 21218
www.press.jhu.edu

Library of Congress Cataloging-in-Publication Data

Names: Jutel, Annemarie, author.
Title: Putting a name to it : diagnosis in contemporary society / Annemarie
    Goldstein Jutel.
Description: Second edition. | Baltimore : Johns Hopkins University Press,
    2024. | Includes bibliographical references and index.
Identifiers: LCCN 2023032544 | ISBN 9781421448923 (paperback) | ISBN
    9781421448930 (ebook)
Subjects: LCSH: Social medicine. | Diagnosis—Social aspects.
Classification: LCC RA418 .J88 2024 | DDC 362.1—dc23/eng/20231219
LC record available at https://lccn.loc.gov/2023032544

A catalog record for this book is available from the British Library.

Special discounts are available for bulk purchases of this book. For more
information, please contact Special Sales at specialsales@jh.edu.

Contents

Acknowledgments

I would like to acknowledge the numerous scholars and colleagues who have helped me to develop my thinking. Most are cited within these pages, from Phil Brown to Sarah Nettleton, Peter Conrad, Allan Horowitz, Robert Aronowitz, and Eviatar Zerubavel. But also the amazing sociologists of diagnosis whose work I have been privileged to read, review, and muse upon, and who have offered feedback on my own: Joanna Kempner, Owen Whooley, Kirsten Barker, Martyn Pickersgill, Susan Kelley, and Mary Ebeling. Thanks also to my clinical friend Lisa Sanders. Closer to home, thanks are due to Kevin Dew. Of course, without my *hoa rangatira*, Thierry Jutel, this book could not have been written.

Some of the material in chapter 3 was previously published in Annemarie Jutel (2017), "Dr. Google" and his predecessors, *Diagnosis* 4 (2):87–91, https://doi.org/10.1515/dx-2016-0045. Some material in chapter 5 was previously published in Annemarie Jutel (2010), Framing disease: The example of female hypoactive sexual desire disorder, *Social Science and Medicine* 70:1084–90, https://doi.org/10.1016/j.socscimed.2009.11.040; and Annemarie Jutel and Barbara Mintzes (2017), Female sexual dysfunction: Medicalizing desire, in *Routledge International Handbook of Critical Mental Health*, edited by Bruce M. Z. Cohen, 162–68. An earlier version of chapter 7 was published in the *Handbook on the Sociology of Health and Medicine*, edited by Alan Petersen (Cheltenham, UK: Edward Elgar, 2023).

Putting a Name to It

What's in a Name?

"Has anyone mentioned Huntington's disease to you?" . . .

Baxter is looking at the ground. Perowne takes his silence as confirmation.

"Do you want to tell me who your doctor is?"

"Why would I do that?"

"We could get you referred to a colleague of mine. He's good. He could make things easier for you."

At this, Baxter turns and angles his head in his attempt to settle the taller man's image on his fovea, that small depression on the retina where vision is most acute. There's nothing anyone can do about a damaged saccadic system. And, generally, there's nothing on offer at all for this condition, beyond managing the descent. But Henry sees now in Baxter's agitated features a sudden avidity, a hunger for information, or hope. Or simply a need to talk.

"What sort of thing?"

"Exercises. Certain drugs."

"Exercise . . ." He snorts on the word. He is right to pick up on the fatuity, the feebleness of the idea. Perowne presses on.

"What has your doctor told you?"   IAN MCEWAN (2004)

The power of the diagnosis is remarkable. Receiving a diagnosis is like being handed a road map in the middle of a forest. It shows the way—but not necessarily the way out. It indicates what the path ahead is going to look like, where it will lead, the difficulty of the climb, and various potential turn-offs. Perhaps it identifies the destination, but not necessarily. With a diagnosis, things don't necessarily get better, but they become clearer. The unexplained becomes explained, and management is defined. Assumptions are made about the future.

The diagnostic moment is simultaneously transformative and contingent. Its transformative power is captured in a story by Ian McEwan, in which Perowne, a neurosurgeon, makes a sidewalk diagnosis of Huntington disease in a thug who is beginning to assault him. The thug's involuntary, uncoordinated, and jerky movements are a dead giveaway. When Perowne names the disorder, his attacker is completely disarmed; the fact of his diagnosis (albeit one he already knew) refocuses the present.

Suzanne Fleischman (1999), in her poignant linguistic discussion of her own (ultimately fatal) disease, explains that "the verbal act of presenting a patient with a diagnosis is never a simple act of conveying value-neutral biomedical information. It is an act fraught with symbolism. If a person is told 'you have cancer' (or any life-threatening disease) *these words* irrevocably alter that person's consciousness, view of the future, relationships with family and friends, and so on. Moreover, the utterance marks a boundary. It serves to divide a life into 'before' and 'after,' and this division is henceforth superimposed onto every rewrite of the individual's life story" (10).

Even in less dramatic circumstances, diagnosis frames reality in significant ways. Few readers of these pages have not had the thought, "What would I do if I found out I had X?"—imagining how life would look if, out of the blue, a serious diagnosis interrupted the quotidian. "Would I even want to know?"

I remember the great ethical debates around *la verité au malade* (telling the truth to patients) when I was a young nursing student in 1980s France. Did health professionals have the right to throw people's lives into disarray by sharing devastating diagnoses with them? Sometimes it was better not to, we were told. I worked at the Clinique Catherine de Sienne—an oncology clinic— where nursing staff were not allowed to pronounce the word "cancer" within earshot of patients. The medical director believed its effect would be too emotionally devastating. We should leave such diagnoses in medical hands, out of respect for their transformative power.* Today, the legal Dispositive d'annonce (the Disclosure Provision) details the prescriptive way in which a serious diagnosis of cancer should be delivered to a patient, surrounded by caution and support. In contrast, when I nursed in medical oncology in the United States for several years, the truth was distributed liberally in its naked, harsh form. In a different culture, rights associated with diagnosis took a different shape. With self-determination at the heart of the American dream, knowledge of one's ailment provides the object against which to react, the starting point for self-realization.

---

* This concern was not new. Thomas Percival discussed it in his 1803 *Medical Ethics*: "Falsehood may lose the essence of lying, and become even praiseworthy," he wrote, "when the adherence to truth is incompatible with the practice of some other virtue of still higher obligation" (1985, 160).

Diagnosis can also be a badge of honor rather than a frightening label to be concealed at all costs. Recognition that diagnosis excuses, explains, justifies, legitimizes, and links individuals in their suffering or in their dysfunction is an important social—rather than clinical—event. The diagnosis is a powerful unifier, one that is highly desired. By virtue of the label, the patient assumes a collective identity and joins new communities. In the case of cancer, the individual may become as much a "battler," or a "survivor," as they become a patient. They may join movements, wearing a ribbon (pink for cancer awareness, purple for Alzheimer's—but also for cystic fibrosis and domestic violence— green for depression, and so on). One poignant example emerges from the overwhelmingly successful Netflix series *Diagnosis*, which is based on putting a name to disorders. This show follows the trajectory of people who do *not* have diagnoses for debilitating conditions; the show crowdsources candidate diagnoses to help. One rapturous fan commented: "Dr Sanders—thank you with every fiber of my being—thank you for doing this. People like my daughter and the families need to know we aren't alone" ("Sarah," October 14, commenting on Gardener 2019). The diagnosis is the unifier, the socializer, the legitimizer.

The contingency of diagnosis, however, is generally not as obvious as its transformative power. Diagnoses are presented as facts of nature, yet they hide a deeply grounded, socially negotiated genesis. As real and observable (and explanatory) as cellular material might be on a glass slide, choosing to look at it (and being able to do so) are contingent on two things: human-made technology and the assumption that particular symptoms are physical. We don't, for example, look for "generosity traits" in blood tests, although nineteenth-century phrenologists and physiognomists sought to confirm their presence in the biophysical.

Diagnosis is always a social creation. That doesn't mean that the diseases it labels aren't "real," but it does mean that before a diagnosis can exist, a condition has to be visible, problematic, and perceived to be related to the field of medicine. All of these factors are linked to social mores. Dyslexia, as one example, may be a disorder in the Western world but not in a nonliterate society. What a particular group perceives to be problematic or unacceptable, needing remedy, is socially contingent. Even something as "real" as COVID-19, in different circumstances, might never have gotten diagnostic status. Imagine if the first cases took place on an isolated farm, and the only people who became ill were young, had light cases, and lacked the opportunity to spread the disease beyond the family. The very real virus would never have come to the attention of medicine and would not have been named. How many diseases never come to broader attention? Never enter a diagnostic manual?

Diagnosis provides a cultural expression of what a given society is prepared to accept as normal and what it believes should be treated. We might lament the fact that witchcraft (Gevitz 2000) and the tendency of "negroes to run away" (drapetomania) (Cartwright 1981) were once seen as diseases, as if we now had a superior understanding of the true nature of medicine. Many readers, however, will remember when "homosexuality" was a disease, classified under code 302 of "sexual deviation" alongside bestiality and pedophilia, but also including transvestitism, fetishism, exhibitionism, and sadomasochism. While it had, in one epoch, been seen as perfectly normal and in another as evidence of moral depravity, its status as a medical concern was solidified by its inscription in the *Diagnostic and Statistical Manual of Mental Disorders (DSM)* as a mental disease (Mendelson 2003).

While witchcraft, drapetomania, and homosexuality bear no relation to medicine's twenty-first-century sensitivity, the knowing lament is misplaced. It's not the technological advancement of medicine that stops us from labeling what we don't like or understand as disease. It's that we can't easily step out of our current vantage point to see the cultural context that historical distance provides.

Might there be similar contemporary examples that will look as droll and as value laden to those who will read our books and diagnostic manuals one hundred years hence? Excited delirium would undoubtedly raise a few eyebrows, as would female hypoactive sexual desire disorder. Excited delirium is a diagnosis that is pronounced most frequently in a coroner's court, when labeling the cause of death of an agitated inmate or patient held under restraint. This syndrome of death in custody ascribes a pathological origin to these suspicious deaths. Medical scapegoat? Genetic fault? Excited delirium deserves careful scrutiny, given the potential it carries for projecting the guilt of overzealous restraint onto pathophysiology (Paquette 2003).

Female hypoactive sexual desire disorder, which I explore in greater depth in chapter 5, might raise the eyebrows of our hypothetical future readers. This diagnosis is applied to women whose lack of sexual desire causes them distress (Clayton et al. 2009). That it exists as a disease category is contingent on unproven beliefs about what constitutes "normal" sexuality. Ah, the elusive "normal"! In other eras, heightened female libido was thought to be an ailment rather than a normative urge because a low sex drive was considered "normal" for women. Psychiatrists used the term "psychopathic" to describe women who engaged in sexual activity beyond the bounds of what genteel society considered moral (Lunbeck 1987).

Diagnoses with social content are not just psychiatric, contested, or controversial. Even mundane and observable conditions such as overweight, infertility, and Lyme disease are dependent for their existence on social judgments and beliefs. I discuss each in greater depth in subsequent chapters, exposing the surprising lack of evidence about the risks of overweight, the nonmedical alternatives to unwanted childlessness, and the convergence of social factors that enabled Lyme disease to be recognized as a disease. As part of this second edition, I also explore the diagnosis that is, at the time of writing, on the tip of everyone's tongue: COVID-19. Even with its now universally recognized and attractively rendered protein spikes (which look, on our pundits' screens, more like a pomander bouquet than a SARS-CoV-2 micrograph), its diagnosis remains a social process, and one worthy of exploration.

Diagnoses are classification tools. They segment and organize the vast continuum of human conditions. Diagnosis validates what counts as disease and what doesn't, prioritizing some conditions over others and always exerting an important material force (Bowker and Star 1999) as it guides medical care. The diagnosis is interpretive and organizational (Balint 1964). When people visit the doctor to find out "what's wrong," they bring a picture of disarray to the consultation: a collection of symptoms and problems they presume to be medical in nature. The diagnosis provides structure—sorting out the real from the imagined, the valid from the feigned, the significant from the insignificant, the physical from the psychological. Once the diagnosis is made, the concordant treatment can be planned, the prognosis reflected on, and resources allocated. Resources include access to such varied items as medications, physiotherapy sessions, sick leave, specialist referrals, and prostheses. The diagnosis is both rudder and anchor: its pursuit guides the individual to the doctor's consulting rooms, while its assignment positions identity and behavior.

Being diagnosed gives permission to be ill. This is what Parsons (1951) referred to as "a claim for exemption." Prior to the recognition of disease, the individual is not "allowed" to fail in their social expectations: getting out of bed and getting dressed, going to work or school, doing housework or looking after the children. Otherwise shortcomings, these "failures" are authorized by the transformative moment of diagnosis. Once diagnosed, the individual is no longer *blamed* for falling short of normative expectations. Instead, they are *treated* (Freidson 1972). The diagnosis enables the individual to socially reintegrate, with allowance made for illness and a sanctioned explanation for their differences.

Because of its power to confirm status and allocate resources, the diagnosis is also an important site of contest and compromise. It is a relational process, with each party (lay and medical) confronting illness with different explanations, understandings, values, and beliefs. The misfit between patient and medical explanatory models may result, individually, in unsatisfactory therapeutic values and goals (Kleinman, Eisenberg, and Good 1978). Or, collectively, it may generate politicization of illness, with social movements and disease advocacy groups battling for recognition, funding, and other forms of support (Brown and Zavestoski 2004).

A Place for a Sociology of Diagnosis?

When I wrote the first edition of this book in 2011, I was making a plea: the time was ripe for a sociology of diagnosis, I argued. Despite the influential role of diagnosis in medicine and in lay-professional relations, it did not have its own sociology, literature, or disciplinary focus. Phil Brown (1990) had called for a sociology of diagnosis many years prior, arguing that diagnosis was only loosely studied by sociologists, notwithstanding the fact that so doing would provide an important insight into how we comprehend disease, health, illness, and the forces that shape our knowledge and practices. The studies that have been made of diagnosis had been more predictably studies of diagnoses—labels in isolation from one another, serving as a heuristic or example of medicalization, disease theory, or history of disease. It's not that diagnosis had been excluded from medical sociology. It's simply that it had been concealed inside these and other areas of focus and hadn't been clearly isolated to be explored on its own. Extirpating diagnosis and revealing it for specific discussion would provide, I argued, an opportunity to study an array of topics from a different perspective: for example, patient-doctor interaction, medicalization, illness experiences, health social movements, disease recognition, and more.

Over the years since the first edition was published, this critical approach to diagnosis, as process and as category, has become far more commonplace. Many erudite scholars have focused their attention on how the sociologist, nay, the critical scholar/citizen, can critique the diagnosis as being something other than purely scientific, value neutral, "the way things are." Darin Weinberg (2020) recently commented that "by insisting the biomedical diagnosis of disease and disability are not innocent of social values, interests, and influences, social constructionism radicalized the explanatory promise of medical sociology . . . [,] biology . . . was recast as diverse forms of socially orchestrated *work* accomplished across a range of historically evolving social institutions" (2).

This second edition, therefore, poses the same questions as before, but with reference to the answers the field has provided in the interim and the supplementary questions it has asked. Emerging fields need to explain what their social warrant is and how they contribute to the broader understandings of the subjects within their remit (Turner 2007).

In the chapters of this book I lay bare the cornerstones of the sociology of diagnosis and what they add to our understandings of medicine in society. As with the first edition, the book does not define the field; rather, it draws together a number of threads that contribute to the critical analysis of health, illness, and disease.

Diagnosis and Medical Identity

The first written use of the term "diagnosis" may have been Thomas Willis, who defined it as "Dilucidation, or Knowledg" in a work published in 1681. He must have used the term previously, as this definition occurs in his posthumous "remaining" works. He had died in 1675. By 1701, George William Lemon referred to "diagnostics [*qui est dignoscendi, peritus*: subtle discerner]": "A knowledge or judgment of the apparent signs of a distemper, or a skill by which the present condition of a distemper is perceived, and this is three-fold, *viz.* 1. A right judgment of the part affected. 2. Of the disease itself. 3. Of its case."

This does not mean that before these writings medical practitioners did not seek to differentiate one ailment from another. Around the time that Willis wrote his definition, changes were afoot in the way medicine considered disease. At the start of the eighteenth century, a classification movement was in full swing, with naturalists from Europe sailing the globe, exploring, collecting, and categorizing the living world. The idea was that taxonomy would provide a mechanism for understanding the earth and for discerning and celebrating God's presence in it. As one mother wrote in a little textbook for her children, "We have reviewed all the classes of beings from insects to man, and we have recognized the hand of God everywhere. We have seen everywhere order and harmony which force our admiration. It would be impossible for us in the face of all these marvels of nature, not to praise He who created all" (*Petites études* 1840, 72).

Medicine followed the natural sciences and engaged in the great classificatory project that would underpin diagnosis. I discuss this further in chapter 2. Classification would identify the features that distinguished one disease from another and the tools by which an individual doctor might assign a particular disease label. It would also offer a means by which the profession could consolidate itself. Classification provided—among other things—the language for discussing matters of collective concern and for passing along medical knowledge.

Just as it provided a focus for medicine to consolidate itself, diagnosis also provided a mechanism for discerning the lay from the professional. Diagnosing is at the base of the social authority afforded the doctor. It sets the doctor apart from the layperson and from other professionals, establishing the doctor's greater knowledge and status (Freidson 1972). Diagnosis also structures relationships within the profession, defining who should assume responsibility for particular disorders (Rosenberg 2002): this complaint to the general practitioner, that one to the immunologist, the hematologist, or the rheumatologist. Particular branches of medicine have used diagnosis to confirm their credibility. Much has been written of the extent to which the *DSM*, psychiatry's bible, became a tool by which the discipline was able to assert its authority at a time when many other professions were encroaching on psychiatry's domain. I discuss this in greater depth in the pages to come.

Diagnoses and their classificatory systems are an important collective arrangement that defines and promotes professional medicine. The authority of medicine, according to de Swaan (1989), resides in such professional agreements about scientific medicine.

At an individual level, the ability to assign a diagnosis also confers power to medicine and its agent, the doctor, as allocator of resources (de Swaan 1989). The diagnosis legitimizes sickness. As discussed previously, when a doctor deems a condition to be medical, the patient receives previously unauthorized privileges, such as permission to be absent from work, priority parking, reimbursement for treatment, or access to services. The doctor certifies the medical nature of the complaint, and "medical advice" informs administrative and policy decisions.

Freidson's (1972) work on professional dominance focuses on the important role of diagnosis in reinforcing medical authority. It is, he postulates, "the . . .

foundation upon which the strength of a profession rests . . . which establishes and supports the profession's claim to honor, income and power. Where illness is the ubiquitous label for deviance in an age, the profession that is custodian of the label is ascendent" (244). He continues: diagnosis is the mission of the doctor, whose task is "to authoritatively label as illness what a complainant suspects to be illness, and also to label as illness what was not previously labeled at all, or what was labelled in some other fashion, under some other institution's jurisdiction" (261).

Authority in medicine comes from its ability to discriminate between behaviors, persons, and conditions, write Peter Conrad and Joseph Schneider (1980). But it also derives from the organization and structure of the medical profession. Medicine has an officially approved monopoly over the right to define health and to treat illness, which results in its high public esteem (Freidson 1972). Doctors, historically, and still today, hold a prominent role in both the health and general social hierarchy, with particular credibility given to their ways of knowing about the body.

Having said this, medical and lay roles are dynamic and currently in flux. Today, access to information once restricted to medical professionals places the layperson in a different position relative to medicine's authority. The expert patient can now discuss, challenge, and contest the medical dominance. In some instances, it must be said, medicine willingly (and perhaps surprisingly) relinquishes ownership of the diagnosis to the patient. For example, a subclassification of migraine in the *International Statistical Classification of Diseases and Related Health Problems 9* was "intractable migraine, *so-stated*" (code 346.11, emphasis added). For this diagnosis to exist, the patient must speak (Bowker and Star 1999). And, during the H1N1 pandemic, diagnostic authority was offered to laypeople in the interest of infection control. Public health messages asked people to stay at home if they had the flu, promoting self-diagnosis of the disease.

The authority to diagnose some medical conditions has also been expanded to include other professional categories. In some countries, a chiropractor or physiotherapist may diagnose certain conditions and prescribe diagnostic technologies, such as X-rays and ultrasounds. Nurse practitioners too may have diagnostic privileges, but both are restricted in the range of diagnoses they may pronounce.

This is not to say that medicine no longer has authority. The biomedical expertise of those trained to practice medicine still carries much weight (Lupton 1997a). The practice of medicine, as well as its authority, is socially contingent and is framed by broader sociotechnological change. Nettleton (2004) discusses this change. She speaks of the informatization of medicine, in which the body is seen as a system of information networks; the art of medicine gives way to evidence-based practice, the physical body defers to the CT scan, information once restricted to medicine is now available to the lay web surfer, and the doctor-patient relationship becomes a meeting of experts. Medicine's jurisdiction is shifting, incorporating new agents and social forces into its contemporary context. The theory of medicalization offers an explanatory framework to understand the changing yet persistent face of medical authority.

Medicalization is the process by which aspects of human existence are assigned to the realm of medicine, to be defined and managed by medicine's authority. Zola (1972) contends that diagnosis plays an important role in medicalization: "If anything can be shown in some way to effect [sic] the workings of the body, and to a lesser extent the mind, then it can be labeled an 'illness' itself or jurisdictionally 'a medical problem'" (495). He marvels at the increasing rate of clinical entities and disorders reported in surveys and studies. This close relationship between medicalization and diagnosis may be the fundamental explanation of why a sociology of diagnosis has not had its own delineation: it has been enveloped in the folds of medicalization.

This broader literature of medicalization informs the sociology of diagnosis by the way it establishes the authoritative and pervasive position of medicine in Western society. Conrad's later definition points to the role of diagnosis in medicalization, indicating the place of illness and disorders in the assertion of medicine's professional territory. But medicalization encompasses more than just diagnosis. For example, infant feeding and child rearing have been—and continue to be—medicalized as part of scientific motherhood (Apple 1995). The privileging of medical authority over other forms of knowledge (even when there is no diagnosis or pathological condition) is notably present in parenting, where the mother or father might seek medical advice for matters of infant health, using medical endorsement for child nutrition and educational products and reading doctor-authored columns or books on childrearing. Similarly, sadness, say, or sexual problems, both arguably nonmedical in nature, are variably transformed by the diagnostic labels "depression" and "erectile dysfunction," triggering an array of medicalized reactions. In these cases, the diagnosis is a specific step into, and an enabling factor of, medicalization.

Understanding medicalization requires us to look at the work of earlier social scientists who were concerned with medicine's authority in contemporary society and its role in legitimizing social concerns (Zola 1983). Before the emergence of the concept of medicalization, Parsons (1951, 1958) and Freidson (1972) discussed the roles of the various components of the social system. Freidson focused particularly on the professional role of the physician with regard to illness, while Parsons explored health and illness in terms of how they affected participation in a social system. "Health and illness," he wrote, "are not only 'conditions' or 'states' of the human individual . . . [;] they are also states evaluated and institutionally recognized in the culture and social structure of societies" (126).

Zola acknowledged that one of the means by which medicalization functions is by affixing diagnostic labels to socially deviant behavior. Peter Conrad explores this in greater depth (1975, 1979, 1992), especially in the book he coauthored with Joseph W. Schneider, *Deviance and Medicalization: From Badness to Sickness* (1980). They note the role of medicine in reform—medical crusaders attempting to influence public morality and behavior—as well as the respect for medical advances. These authors propose a five-stage model by which a deviant behavior is medicalized through diagnoses: defining the behavior as deviant, discovering the behavior from within the medical community, making claims, challenging the existing designation to bring the behavior to medical turf, and institutionalizing the behavior via diagnosis.

A number of scholars focus on the myriad of social conditions receiving medical attention and diagnostic labels. John Rosecrance (1985) extends Conrad and Schneider's model to his work on compulsive gambling. Scholars have explored hyperactivity (P. Conrad 1975), alcoholism (Blaxter 1978), menstruation (Smith-Rosenberg and Rosenberg 1973; Vertinsky 1994), pregnancy (Barker 1998), sexuality (Tiefer 1996), obesity (Jutel 2008), andropause (P. Conrad 2007), adult attention-deficit/hyperactivity disorder (ADHD) (P. Conrad 1979), male infertility (Hanna and Gough 2020), autism spectrum disorder (Chiri, Bergey, and Mackie 2022), and even compulsive buying (Lee and Mysyk 2004). These are all examples of the transfer of life events and ways of being to the auspices of medical care.

That a particular condition should find itself assigned to medicine for its management rather than in a place it had previously been located, may be variably assessed with skepticism, with relief, or with wonder. The critique of medicalization is most frequently one of "it oughtn't to be"; the particular condition would be better managed by the midwife, the priest, the prison guard.

That the problem should be diagnosed and medically managed is a kind of medical imperialism, a step too far: the medicalization of childbirth (Brubaker and Dillaway 2009), of sexuality (Jutel 2010a; Jutel and Mintzes 2017), of menstruation (Mamo and Fosket 2009). Riding on the coattails of diagnosis, numerous industries fan the flame of medicalization to sell their wares. Clarke and her colleagues (2003) have referred to the *bio*medicalization of society: "Health itself and the proper management of chronic illnesses are becoming individual moral responsibilities to be fulfilled through improved access to knowledge, selfsurveillance, prevention, risk assessment, the treatment of risk, and the consumption of appropriate self-help/biomedical goods and services" (162).

One interesting example of diagnostification is intersex. The complex problem of sexual ambiguity at birth caused many problems for young people, whose families and doctors believed that the condition needed to be "resolved" before the child had consciousness of their sex or gender. Drastic and irreversible corrective therapies were undertaken ruthlessly and often mistakenly. If intersex were a diagnosis, pondered its advocates, would clinicians then follow guidelines rather than rush to mismeasured therapeutics? Medicalization was thus undertaken as a chosen project, to benefit individuals—albeit individuals who did believe themselves not to be ill but rather in need of a more moderate medicine, rendered docile via diagnosis (Davis 2015).

The expansion of diagnostic categories is not without risk and can have severe iatrogenic results. The treatment that accompanies a diagnosis may expose an individual to undesirable or unintended secondary effects. As one example, the medicalization of shyness, which results in the diagnoses of social phobia, social anxiety disorder, and avoidant personality disorder, encourages patients to request, and doctors to recommend, pharmaceutical remedies, some of which have resulted in reports of devastating side effects (S. Scott 2006). As I note in chapter 5, this focus on diagnosis provides a fertile ground for the commercial exploitation of patients and doctors alike.

Diagnosis and Lay Identity

While diagnosis might arrange and consolidate the identity of the professional, it is more likely to *rearrange* individual identity, threatening previous self-definition as the individual now "inhabits" an illness (Klinkenborg 1994, 79). For the person who has a serious or chronic disease, "illness becomes a trope for new attitudes toward the self; it also influences perceptions of that self by others, including, notably, employers and insurers" (Fleischman 1999, 13).

An individual narrative of disease is not, however, independent of the *regime* associated with a diagnosis, proposes Klawiter (2008). A disease regime is the cultural, spatial, and historical practices associated with a diagnosis, and it goes beyond the circumstances of the individual and the physiological nature of the illness. Klawiter demonstrates how the narrative of one individual altered over time, as a result of different cultural conditions in which she experienced two separate diagnoses of breast cancer. The agendas, identities, social relations, policies, and emotional vocabularies embodied in different "regimes of practice" around breast cancer transformed public discourses and other forms of cultural production and in turn transformed the narrative of the individual.

Diagnosis may also create collective identities, removing the individual from the isolation of their suffering and providing new potential networks of support. In turn, this collective identity has political potential to shape, and in some cases challenge, professional authority, political imperatives, and social identity (Brown and Zavestoski 2004). Phil Brown (1995) has written about how diagnosis offers a tool for political engagement. Diagnoses such as posttraumatic stress disorder, black lung, and environmental disease offer social recognition for victims of abuse or toxic exposure, opening the door to care and to compensation.

Collective identity may be virtual. A growing number of internet communities are focused on diagnoses. Web pages play a part in the social health movement, gathering individuals around both existing and emerging diseases. Dumit (2006) explains that internet communities offer a means of survival for those who have medically unexplained symptoms. They provide an alternative support structure when the absence of diagnosis impugns the medical legitimacy of the individual's complaint.

Increasingly, the pressure of these social support structures contributes to the creation of diagnostic categories. Long COVID is one such example, according to Callard and Perego (2021). It is a diagnosis, they argue, borne of collective suffering and social media communities. Through Twitter, #LongCovid assumed an increasingly influential presence in the public and, subsequently, medical consciousness. Progressively, it gained purchase and disrupted conventional pathways for disease recognition.

In any case, the question of identity—which diagnosis (or its absence) helps to consolidate—is important in the social context of health, illness, and disease. It is at the base of lay health movements, it infiltrates doctor-patient relationships, it is part of how individuals make sense of their illness and its impact on their day-to-day experiences, and it is a way of belonging for many who find their conditions marginalizing them in untenable ways.

An Avenue for Understanding

Medicine is temporally situated, and it makes its diagnoses on the basis of the technology and values available at a given time. As an unidentified writer wrote in the *British Medical Journal* in 1886, "The imperfection of our medical vocabulary is not a matter for surprise. It is the measure and gauge of the imperfection of our medical knowledge, and only perfect knowledge admits of a perfect nomenclature" (*British Medical Journal* 1886, 1116).

Ivan Illich contends that "disease always intensifies stress, defines incapacity, imposes inactivity, and focuses apprehension on nonrecovery, on uncertainty, and on one's dependence upon future medical findings." He continues: "Once a society organizes for a preventative disease-hunt, it gives epidemic proportions to diagnosis. This ultimate triumph of therapeutic culture turns the independence of the average healthy person into an intolerable form of deviance" (1976, 104).

Goode writes in a similar tone, pointing out that "by devising a linguistic category with specific connotations, one is designing the armaments for a battle; by having it accepted and used, one has scored a major victory" (1969, 89). The power of the diagnosis is its classificatory functions: the diagnosis does the work of "making it appear that science describes nature (and nature alone) and that politics is about social power (and social power alone)" (Bowker and Star 1999, 46). The work of the diagnosis is often invisible, however, "erased by [its] naturalization into the routines of life," concealing conflict and multiplicity beneath layers of obscure representation (47).

Most readers of this book have, at some point, gone to see the doctor to "find out what's wrong." Some go with trepidation, wondering whether they're wasting the doctor's time ("It's probably nothing"), while others leave with even more unease than when they went in ("If nothing's wrong with me, why do I feel this way?"). Yet a third group leaves a consultation with a clear sense of what is remiss, instructions about treatment, and, with some luck, an anticipation of when and how the ailment will resolve. Diagnosis structures the reality of individuals, as it clarifies and sometimes explains what they experience. Interactions in the doctor's rooms are strongly framed by what it means both to be a patient and to be a doctor. Subservience to medical authority is both reassuring and problematic. Good patients show signs of "compliance" with and "adherence" to doctor's orders. Informed self-advocates work hard with, and sometimes against, the doctor, probing and questioning why their complaint is or isn't considered medical and protesting if a psychogenic cause is proposed: less physical, less real.

In today's world, where information abounds, the diagnostic relationship between patient and doctor has changed. Patients may, at odds with Balint's description, propose a diagnosis rather than an ailment when they consult. Or they may circumvent the doctor altogether. They calculate their body mass index, take depression self-tests, or use medical terminology to describe their idiosyncrasies and those of their friends. "Are you sure you don't have ADD?" they might quiz, even able to use a readily recognizable acronym for attention deficit disorder. Laypeople are changing the shape of what diagnosis means in practice.

The "modern" patient is the ideal: an informed "consumer" who can sit on an equal platform with the doctor as a result of now-open access to information previously restricted to the medical profession. The idealized clinical encounter is a cooperative interaction that brings patient and doctor together in a kind of handshake agreement about what ails the former and what the latter can do in response. It is not always so simple, particularly as the encounter is about far more, as Hunter (1991) points out, than a simple classification of our malady; focusing on the diagnosis draws attention away from the care of the person who is ill. Furthermore, the profession's acknowledgments of its limitations, as well as of myriad social influences on its classificatory practices, needs attention from within.

Exploring the social forces that influence the clinical process of diagnosis provides a greater understanding of both the fluidity and the fallibility of the diagnosis. Diagnoses do not exist ontologically. They are concepts that bind the biological, the technological, the social, the political, and the lived. Thomas Laqueur asserts that "believing is seeing." Despite the advent of autopsy and a presumed clear vision of the ways structures were connected, Renaissance anatomists still depicted the vagina as an inside-out penis and menstrual flow as transformed into breast milk during lactation (Laqueur 1990). Similarly, diagnosis captures what the medical institution currently believes to be "the way things are." Suffice it to say, the world of facts is not detachable from an a priori conceptual framework.

Sociology of diagnosis is an important avenue for understanding not only lay experience of illness and lay-professional discord, as I discussed above, but also patient compliance, disease control, public health, health education, and many other aspects of health and illness. Kleinman and colleagues' claims of thirty years ago hold strong today: understanding social science is necessary to deal competently with essential nonbiomedical aspects of clinical practice. They maintain that medicine is both a biological and a social science (Kleinman, Eisenberg, and Good 1978). Focusing on both social and biological aspects assists clinicians in treating patients as well as diseases, a sometimes neglected feature of contemporary medical practice (see A. Goldstein 2007; Leder 1990). Understanding the social frames within which diagnoses are generated and grasping the impact of the label is clinically powerful. As Aronowitz (2001) cautions, there is an "essential continuity between persons who have symptoms that have been given a name and disease-like status and persons whose suffering remains unnamed and unrecognized" (808).

Sociology of diagnosis has a salient role in understanding health, illness, and disease: unpacking and identifying the play of interests that enter into discussions of what priorities should be set and what goals attained. Diagnosis defines the field of medicine and its professional reach, serves as the nexus in which the clinical encounter takes place, arbitrates normality and difference, organizes a patient's illness, and determines how resources are allocated. In this introduction I have, with a broad brush, covered a range of considerations that contribute to a sociology of diagnosis: the place of naming in medicine and the tensions naming can engender. But there is more work to be done. A rich collection of structures, agents, and actions enters into the diagnostic arena and deserves consideration. Identifying, analyzing, and understanding them and their connections will ultimately contribute to a better understanding of medicine's goals and who performs them, as well as the relationship of medicine to culture and society.

CHAPTER ONE

Lumping or Splitting

Classification in Medical Diagnosis

> We are not to suppose that there are only a certain number of divisions
> in any subject, and that unless we follow these, we shall divide it wrongly
> and unsuccessfully: on the contrary every subject is as it were all joints,
> it will divide wherever we choose to strike it, and therefore according to
> our particular object at different times we shall see fit to divide it very
> differently. THOMAS ARNOLD (1839)

Diagnosis is one of medicine's most powerful classification tools. Understanding classification must be part of the quest to understand the social context and implications of diagnosis more clearly. Classification provides a foundation for the recognition and study of illness: deciding how the vast expanse of nature can be partitioned into meaningful chunks, stabilizing and structuring what is otherwise disordered. The classifications into which doctors and laypeople slot their explanations of illness determine much about disease. Yet little is revealed about how these classifications are produced, the principles involved, the voices present and interests satisfied, or those silenced and disappointed.

Effective classification recognizes difference as well as similarity. By classifying, we are putting items together that have more in common with one another than they do with things we have decided belong in another category (Zerubavel 1996). There needs to be a reasonable rationale for placing similar objects together, enough resemblance among members of the category for them to be associated, while not obfuscating difference. This is the principle of Ockham's razor: "Entities are not to be multiplied beyond necessity" (*Entia non sunt multiplicanda praeter necessitatem*) (Ockham 1997). Ockham's principle highlights simplicity: don't get too complex when a few general categories will do.

But the rationale for classifying is always fluid, as Arnold signals: subjects are "all joints," he says, pointing out that the "various branches of human knowledge are capable of the most different arrangements according to the light in which we wish to regard them" (1839, 5–6).

Arnold used "the vegetable creation" to describe the opportunistic nature of classification. If we are to classify vegetables in relation to people, he explained, we might put wheat, potatoes, and figs in the same conceptual basket. These are all products of the vegetable kingdom that are *edible* for humans. On the contrary, if we are concerned with their botanical taxonomy, the classification changes: grasses, tubers, and trees become the organizing principles of these clusters. We'll put wheat and flax together, potatoes and deadly nightshade, fig trees and oaks.

Similar fluidity is present in medicine's classifications. Ailments may be grouped according to how or why the information needs to be processed, by location of symptoms, their treatment, the threat they present to public health, their etiology, their prognosis, how much they cost to cure, and so on. While one could lump the common cold with COVID-19 as a result of the similarity of their causative agents (both coronaviruses), from a public health perspective, the classification is not so useful. There would be more sense in grouping Ebola, influenza, and COVID-19, despite their viral dissimilarities—because of their contagion and public impact.

To classify a disease, it must first be visible to medicine. This visibility is not based simply on technology: being able to distinguish a particular microbe or genetic translocation. Rather, such recognition requires differentiation between the idiosyncratic and the generalizable. Do one person's fever and achy joints have anything to do with another's? If they don't, they're more likely to remain unfiled and unclassified: not a disease but an individual expression of something yet to be understood. The example of Lyme disease is helpful to understanding this question of visibility. Lyme disease was recognized in the mid-1970s. It was not hard to name and was easy to identify, as there was a clear infectious agent at the source of the disease with a specific vector, a tick-borne spirochete. Despite the tangibility and empirical evidence of its existence, it was not easily visible. The low-grade fever, headache, malaise, and joint pain of its sufferers could easily have been the result of any one of a number of systemic, infectious processes. It was the clustering of cases within a geographic region and in a particular time frame that foregrounded this particular condition as a discrete entity worthy of research and for which a causative agent had to be sought. A number of Connecticut mothers (from the area around the town of Lyme) brought the cluster to the attention of public health officials. Had the cases been more geographically dispersed, the sufferers less articulate, or public health officers less receptive to its description as a unified condition, it might not have been named (Aronowitz 1998).

A diagnosis must not only be visible but also agreed on. There is a difference between presuming links between particular groups of symptoms and including the diagnosis in medical taxonomy. AIDS is a case in point. While we might have a clear picture of what AIDS is today—an acquired immune deficiency syndrome resulting from infection by the human immunodeficiency virus—the condition went through many previous configurations. Initially, it was the opportunistic infections typical of AIDS that were considered as the disease problem: clustered observations of pneumocystis carinii pneumonia and Kaposi sarcoma in particular populations (gay men, hemophiliacs, Haitians, and heroin users as well as those who had sexual relations with people from these groups). Many causative factors were evoked, including fungi, allergies, and chemicals. The isolation and identification of HIV and agreement on its contribution to the observed immunodeficit did not occur until 1984 (Gallo and Montagnier 2003).

Deciding what warrants grouping into categories and what needs to be seen as idiosyncratic and isolated—just one person's sickness—is part of how diagnosis organizes and directs medicine and public health (and is the challenge embodied in Ockham's razor). At an individual level, the clinician will classify the patient complaint, assessing symptoms for characteristics that bring to mind a particular pathology, a previous case, a textbook memory. Collectively, classification of diseases validates, locates, and distributes: designating whether a disease is real, if it is psychological or physical, under what subdisciplinary jurisdiction it falls, what treatment it requires, how many resources should be assigned to it, and so on.

Ultimately, the goal of classification is to simplify. Recognizing the similarity among conditions in order to group them provides a basis for communication, for logical connection, for research, and for statistical analysis. For a problem to be counted as a condition, it must first be identified as "the same as" or "different from" another; if different, the distinction between the two must be clear—or at least rational. As Arnold's "joints" illustrate, distinctions can be made in any of a number of places. Zerubavel (1991) uses a contrasting metaphor, describing nature as a continuum broken up as we see fit. Both positions underline the fact that to classify is to reify. Diagnosis is the *making real* of conceptual categories.

Speaking of the "conceptualization" of disease is not to suggest that diseases do not exist. It is rather to point out *how* they come to exist. A disease might be conceptualized on the basis of its causation. For example, dengue fever is an infectious disease caused by one of four dengue viruses. It may result in bleeding disorders and a skin rash; despite these features, it is not conceptualized as either hematological or dermatological.

Disease conceptualization can be based on location in the body (meningitis or pneumonia) or on symptoms (migraine or asthma). And diseases may be reconceptualized on the basis of new knowledge and understandings. A blood disorder referred to in the nineteenth century as chlorosis, over its history passed through numerous configurations on the basis of identity politics, laboratory techniques, and therapeutic approaches, confirms that there is no timelessness about disease, and technology cannot confirm all (Wailoo 1997).

In this chapter, I explore the aims of classification in general and their embodiment in medical diagnosis, using liberal historical examples of the diagnostic project. Classification schemas serve as archives of the practical politics of medicine (Blaxter 1978; Bowker and Star 2000; P. Brown 1995). From John Graunt's seventeenth-century *Reflections on the Weekly Bills of Mortality* to the 10th and still-current revision of the *International Statistical Classification of Diseases and Related Health Problems* (ICD), these nosologies highlight changes in medical models, legislation, and belief systems as much as they do the changes in medical knowledge. But mainly I will focus on why we classify in medicine: the rationale for splitting illness into different categories and the political and social compromises that these categories conceal.

The Aims of Classification

To classify is to arrange things in groups that are divided from one another by clear boundaries (Durkheim and Mauss 1903). Classification determines the response or reaction we should have in the presence of one group of objects (or conditions) as opposed to another (Hayes and Adams 2008). Seeking to understand classification and how it operates is not a new concern. Aristotle's doctrines of categories were the backbone of his philosophical inquiry. Aristotle presented a "schema of things" that accounted for both the particular and the universal (Novak 1965).

Aristotle's classification is hierarchical. The highest level on this hierarchy is the category, of which there are 10: substance, quantity, quality, relatives, somewhere, sometime, being in a position, having, acting, and being acted on. Each category contains a range of differentiated "species," which themselves may be further divided into genera. The point at which no further differentiation takes place is where the "particular" of a species finally sits at the lowest level. The category starts at the most general, branching progressively down to the lowest level, where the individual substances, such as "this man" or "that horse," are found (M. Cohen 2008).

Many centuries later, in 1837, William Farr echoed Aristotle's intent, couching the importance of the universal in scientific terms. He referred to classification as "a method of generalization" whose value was in its ability to serve as basis for empirical research, to "facilitate . . . inquiries and . . . yield general results" (qtd. in WHO 1957, viii).

Classification theorists have postulated a number of aims of classification. These include (among other things) organizing knowledge (Jacob 1992); developing a useful description of a sample and discovering unsuspected but potentially important clusterings (Fleiss et al. 1971); achieving stable and predictive classes (Silvestri and Hill 1964); and perhaps above all, as Richardson wrote at the beginning of the past century, reducing a disorderly mass to an orderly whole (E. Richardson 1901).

Classifying is at the heart of how we understand the world. It is, according to Zerubavel (1991), the means by which we bestow meaning on things and concepts around us. It creates the "diagnostic niches" into which we place what we feel, see, smell, eat, and so forth. It is how we explain our experience of life and how we partition the social world.

Robert Sokal (1974) describes classification as having three aims. While his at-the-time novel approach to classification in the natural sciences (numerical taxonomy) was not universally accepted and has since been superseded by other methods, the aims he describes provide a succinct summary, useful for understanding disease classification. Reminiscent of Aristotle's desire to see the individual in the general, Sokal attributes to classification the following purposes: streamlining memory by grouping individual cases into representative groups, determining relationships between the members of one category and those of another, and generating questions about how the order that a classificatory system embodies has come to be. Classifications should help us to think about nature efficiently, he explains: "The world is full of single cases: single individuals of animal or plant species, single case histories of disease, single books, rocks or industrial concerns. By grouping numerous individual objects into a taxon the description of the taxon subsumes the individual descriptions of the objects contained within it" (185).

Classification also seeks to create meaningful juxtapositions to or interfaces between groups of objects. Classification can only be about isolated, bounded boxes if there is something beyond the boundary. It is part of a system in which one category sits in relation to what it isn't. The system makes generalizations about constituent objects feasible and meaningful, such that an object classified as X is not Y, or is mainly not Y and is more reasonably X. Nonidentical items may thus sit in same classificatory categories. For example, cows and people are both animals, despite having different numbers of legs, while cows and chairs, despite both having four legs, are unlikely to be found in the same category (Sokal 1974).

Classification aims to be heuristic (Sokal 1974). A classification provides a hypothesis from which investigation into the perceived order can take place, be tested, and provide insight into etiological, social, and pragmatic explanations for the system of categorization. Systems to describe nature are dynamic; the best means for classifying objects (conditions) are constantly evolving as new explanatory frameworks, causative factors, and idiosyncratic presentations come to the fore.

Classification of Diseases

Classifying disease (diagnosis) has many intended purposes that serve both medical and lay interests. Some of these purposes serve both interests simultaneously, and others are more specifically linked with one group or the other. From providing a common language for discussing diseases to creating personal and collective identity, diagnostic classification organizes other activities beyond any immediate therapeutic goal. I review in the next few pages some of the primary goals of disease classification.

Clearly, diagnosis is the foundational step in determining the appropriate therapy for what ails an individual. Indeed, seeking treatment often leads the pursuit of diagnosis. By identifying the disease, one is a step closer to identifying a concordant treatment and cure. When a cure is not available, at least a prognosis may be agreed on. With a sense of what to expect from a particular condition—how things may progress—it may be easier to accept one's sort.

Engelhardt (1992) explains, "One invests labor in making a diagnosis not simply in order to know truly, but because one would hope to be able to avoid or mitigate some unpleasant state of affairs. In the case of prognosis, one wants at least to be able to plan for likely unpleasant future developments" (73).

When a condition is diagnosed, a different range of remedies becomes available. Think of the diagnosis of infertility. From a nonmedical perspective, it could be described simply as the state of unwanted childlessness (Becker and Nachtigall 1992). As a disease, however, it gains access to an entire new arsenal of potential remedies. It becomes worthy of medicine's attention and warrants medical solutions. Arguably, infertility is not a disease in the sense that it causes no physical distress to its sufferers. It is not accompanied by gastric upset or sore joints. It may make people suffer nonetheless, distressed by the undesirable social condition of unintended childlessness. But it can be diagnosed and treated. A range of infertility treatments including hormonal manipulation, acute monitoring of cervical or sperm function, and in vitro fertilization simultaneously redefine this social problem and replace its social solutions. As a nonmedical condition, unwanted childlessness is remedied in other ways. Changing aspirations (say, refocusing desire on other aspects of life) and adopting or fostering children are legitimate social approaches to resolving the distress. Such actions, however, are "are apparently viewed as more undesirable once a biomedical approach is initiated because they symbolize a dual failure: the failure to conceive and the failure to be cured" (Becker and Nachtigall 1992, 468).

Diagnosis also serves an important didactic and communicative role in medicine. This is in contrast to ancient medicine. Ancient Greek medicine, according to historian Ilza Veith (1981), did not have a medical terminology. "So long as medical knowledge was restricted, a narrative descriptive style was used to evoke a picture of a disease, where nowadays one word, a simple disease name, would suffice" (221). Developing a nomenclature would lead to working therapy, which in turn would enable communication between doctors and allow medicine to be more efficient in its tasks (Fischer-Homberger 1970). Thomas Sydenham is generally credited as the father of classificatory medicine, committed to naming disease in order to advance the field by enabling communication between doctors and between doctors and students.

"All diseases then ought to be reduc'd to certain and determinate kinds, with the same exactness as we see it done by botanic writers in their treatises of plants," he wrote. His goal was "the improvement of physick" (Sydenham 1742, iv). Fisher-Homberger (1970) recounts that Sydenham, and his good friend John Locke, threw themselves at nosology in a kind of despair. Medicine was not terribly successful in its task, and resignation, laced with hope, about the state of the field prompted them to consider that by engaging in this systematic classification of disease types, they might find that medicine could make strides toward improving survival. "I am persuaded," wrote Sydenham, "that there never will be any great and considerable advances made in the art of *healing*, till all hypotheses and mechanical reasoning are out of vogue, and till men are come about again to the antient method of experiment, and the common obvious reasoning entire from thence" (1742, vii).

According to Fisher-Homberger (1970), "Two notions of beginners in medicine on the one hand and medicine herself as a beginner on the other tend to overlap. It is true that the nosological systems were designed to help medical students, but they were also to further medicine as a science, for as such it had still not progressed beyond its initial stages. For centuries it had kept going astray. Its language had become confused and unintelligible. There had to be a radically new approach to it. Nosology provided a possible new approach and its terminology provided the linguistic means to deal with it" (400).

As recently as the mid-twentieth century, the limitations of the language of medicine were observed by Michael Balint (1964), who explains the need for better diagnostic terminology in psychiatry: "This want of a proper language is one reason for the unsatisfactory and often irritating lack of understanding between the general practitioner and the psychiatric consultant. We psychiatrists cannot yet give the general practitioners the badly needed set of technical terms which they could use confidently and which would help them to understand the deeper personality problems of their patients. For the time being our descriptions of pathological states are vague, complicated, longwinded, easily misunderstood when not backed by lengthy explanations" (40).

Disease identification and naming has been an important part of psychiatry's professional project, as I illustrate in the pages to come. The development and revisions of the *Diagnostic and Statistical Manual of Mental Disorders* (DSM) were to provide a uniform language to discuss mental illness and transform diagnostic categories that brought psychiatry more in line with its medical counterdisciplines, shifting psychotherapy away from the purview of physicians, creating opportunities for clinical research, and favoring psychophar-macology (Mayes and Horwitz 2005).

Diagnosis continues to be at the heart of medical education, serving both as objective and as heuristic. Medical textbooks are organized around disease types, with physiology and biology introduced and explained via disease categories. Disease principles and specific diseases organize how medical students learn about the body.

Diagnosis enables research about disease. Research takes place when like can systematically be described as like, testing treatment efficacy empirically, making generalizations about disease patterns, and understanding causes of illness and death. The first disease classification document was devoted to this aim. In 1662, John Graunt published the *Natural and Political Observations* [. . .] *made upon the Bills of Mortality*, an epidemiological document studying where and when particular groupings of causes of death could be found. Graunt's publication sought to predict disease trends. He observed that people tended only to look at the bottom line ("the foot") of the weekly bills of mortality—namely, how many people died. He felt that much greater use could be made of this information to protect the population. The bills could predict the frequency and proportion of "sickly years," the relationship between "healthfull and frutifull seasons," the difference between "City and Country air, &c." (37). He made strong representation for a more detailed and standardized classification of causes of death, which would provide information about the diseases of the kingdom. While the plague figured prominently in social consciousness, Graunt argued that to understand its impact, it had to be carefully distinguished from other diseases that "forerun the plague a Year, two or three" (34) and compounded the mortality statistics.

Graunt's work had no design on medical education; rather, it was published to identify mortality trends and extrapolate either remedial or palliative measures to enhance survival. This analysis, clearly, sought a social frame. "The observations which I happened to make (for I designed them not) upon the Bills of Mortality, have fallen out to be both Political, and Natural, some concerning Trade, and Government, others concerning the Air, countries, Seasons, Fruitfulness, Health, Diseases, Longevety, and the proportions between the Sex, and Ages of Mankind."

Graunt wrote the above in 1662 as he presented his observations on the Bills of Mortality to Sir Robert Moray of the Privy Council to King James (Graunt 1662b). This early classification of diseases presented arguments for the recording of "accompts of Burials, and Christenings [to be] kept universally, and now called for, and perused by Magistrate."

The original *International Classification of Diseases (ICD)*, which I discuss further in the following section, followed Graunt's tradition of attempting to understand the causes of death in order to summarize and describe trends in mortality that could help direct public health initiatives and policy. Diagnosis thus enables statistical analysis of disease and mortality by providing categorical units for synthesis. This type of analysis can extend, however, far beyond simply recording mortality trends. Counting illnesses as diagnostic units enables many different kinds of measurements. Medical record review, quality outcomes, financial expenditure, and risk assessments use diagnosis to assess, measure, and predict what factors lead to which diseases, how much these diseases cost, and the results of their treatment. Deciding how much to reimburse for particular kinds of care; where to concentrate public health efforts; who is at risk from what; and how particular communities, organizations, or professionals "rank" in terms of successful treatment of various diseases—all this relies on the diagnostic unit.

Similarly, the evidence-based practice (EBP) paradigm relies on diagnosis. Its fundamental premise is one of decision making based on the generalizability of scientific findings. Without diagnostic categories, we could not systematically appraise the empirical evidence upon which EBP is constructed. Grounded in epidemiological understandings of illness and therapeutic efficacy, EBP uses diagnoses and their associated signs, symptoms, and treatment as the specific targets for intervention and appraisal.

A clinical diagnosis, with its inherent biomedical justification, contributes to sickness identity, both individual and collective. Susan Sontag (1978) describes illness as the "night-side of life, a more onerous citizenship. Everyone who is born holds that citizenship, in the kingdom of the well and in the kingdom of the sick. Sooner or later each of us is obliged, at least for a spell, to identify ourselves as citizens of that other place" (3). By recognizing the "other place," the newly diagnosed emerges from the isolation of their private disease, locating new networks of support but also a transformed identity. The individual illness fits into a wider explanation that may include many other individuals with similar, or at least related, complaints. It also offers the potential for politicized collective illness identity (Brown et al. 2004).

Klawiter's work on breast cancer speaks eloquently to how diagnosis (specifically breast cancer) creates both individual and collective identity (Klawiter 1999). In the mid-1980s, cancer became a movement, with its advocates, its survivors, and its campaigns. By the early 1990s, *breast* cancer inspired a specific social movement of its own with a variety of politicized identities with which women variably identified. These identities were not uniform; Klawiter describes three. The first revolves around honor and survival. It casts medicine as the savior and early detection as an important weapon in the battle to beat breast cancer. This identity is linked to normative femininity and courage. It uses fighting words and celebrates those who have vanquished the disease. Klawiter describes the pink-beribboned breast cancer survivor as "proudly, voluntarily, and publicly mark[ing] herself . . . visually embodying an identity not otherwise apparent. This is an act of social disobedience-a collective 'coming out,' a rejection of stigma and invisibility, and a simultaneous appropriation of the traditional color of femininity for the survivor identity" (111). An alternative to this identity is one that mobilizes against biomedicine, emphasizing the inequalities inherent in the system and the biased focus on heteronormativity. It promotes activism and social services. Finally, a feminist environmental justice movement casts breast cancer as the result of a toxic global cancer industry with interests in promoting as therapeutic the carcinogenic chemicals that are at the root of the disease. In this case, the person who has breast cancer is a victim, fighting the pharmaceutical industry, whose focus is on profit, whatever the human cost.

The ability of the diagnosis to convey identity is powerful. Patients who refer to themselves as "diabetic" or "bipolar" incorporate the disease as part of the self via the syntactic construction of being: I *am* diabetic. Becoming the diagnosis, being replaced by it, is reinforced by synecdoche (taking the part for the whole), common among the conversations of attendant health professionals. "Can you check on the MI [myocardial infarction] in room 3?" The patient, summed up as this disease or that body part, becomes subsumed by what was only part of who they were before (Fleischman 1999).

The transformative nature of the diagnostic moment may tell us we are sick even before we are ill and provides us with a clear message about who we are. Things will never be the same again: "In a person suffering severe or chronic illness, just as in a community suffering an epidemic, disease provokes a crisis of self-definition; internal boundaries shift, and the complex structures of identity rearrange themselves" (Klinkenborg 1994, 78).

Certain diagnoses have mythic significance for the identity of their sufferers. Tuberculosis was held to selectively attack the romantic exile, the artist:

both passionate and passive. It was considered a mark of breeding and of culture (Star and Bowker 1997). One nineteenth-century husband wrote of his wife, "She has that ardent pallor which we have always dreamt about and which devours our hearts. On her dull skin, light dances in a violet and greenish glow. Her teeth shine like those of a young tigress, and her eyes have a strange gleam which frightens me" (qtd. in Bricart 1985, 182–83). Melancholy was similarly long held as a badge of honor, the mark of "all truly outstanding men with creative and moral qualities," according to Aristotle (qtd. in Melechi 2003, 13). The "melancholick" had a particularly elevated social status over the populace, who were more likely to be afflicted with mundane grief, or the mopes (Melechi 2003).

The multiple purposes of diagnostic classification—treatment and prognosis, medical education and communication, research, and identity—are enacted by the classification systems used by medicine and by the lay pursuit of diagnosis to organize the experience of illness. I briefly review two important diagnostic systems used in Western medicine, the *ICD* and the *DSM*, before concluding this chapter with a commentary on how values and political actions become embedded in and reproduced by diagnostic classifications.

Classification Systems

Prominent contemporary disease classificatory documents such as the *ICD* and the *DSM* start with a historical genealogy, highlighting other statistical and nosological precedents. The influence of, and deference to, history is an interesting feature of contemporary medical classification. As Blaxter (1978) explained, medical classifications are perhaps best considered as a "museum of past and present concepts of the nature of disease" (10). Phil Brown (1995) adds that contemporary classification systems contain vestiges of many prior conceptions of disease, as distant as eighteenth-century botanical classification or later clinical pathology, as well as a number of other models, some no longer explicitly present in practice but still firmly ingrained in the classification system.

Were disease more like library books, one could impose an external constraint on how and in which section conditions would be filed, and it would simply be a matter of allocating a particular condition to a given classification, creating a logical rationale for the cases of slightly looser fit. But medicine has, according to Blaxter (1978), built its classification system by identifying its parts first before the whole, thus creating a structure that bears the indelible imprint of its antecedents.

This back-to-front approach to a system is not surprising—or even avoidable. Changes in medical theory, technological ability, or values are frequent enough that they cannot give rise to new classifications systems at each turning point. That such changes lead to remodeling rather than reconstruction is evident in the presence of eponymous diagnoses that hearken back to their historical origins (Blaxter 1978), such as Raynaud, Down, and Graves syndromes.

International Statistical Classification of Diseases and Related Health Problems

The *ICD* is a diagnostic classification system published by the World Health Organization (WHO). Its presence infiltrates medical bureaucracy, if not medical practice. It is used to collect and compare morbidity and mortality statistics around the world. The *ICD* is part of a suite of classifications published by the WHO, including also *International Classification of Functioning, Disability and Health* and the *International Classification of Health Interventions*. All of these classification systems have been negotiated and approved by the WHO member countries and are used for international comparisons and reporting (WHO 2023b).

The *ICD* is what Bowker (1996) refers to as an "information infrastructure." It is embedded in myriad databases, supports medical work, has international reach, is learned as part of membership in the medical profession, and is linked with numerous conventions (50). Its purpose and shape are grounded in an information-gathering practice that is defined by nations anxious to understand, support, and monitor their citizenry. What makes the *ICD* interesting as a medical classification document is its genesis in politics of the state. Classification is an important mechanism by which the modern state may promote its political and economic functioning, central to which is protecting the health and longevity of its citizens (52). The *ICD* was developed as a response to nineteenth-century epidemics, which themselves were only enabled by modern imperialists who could get from place to place more quickly than in the past, carrying a germ with them. This meant that the bacillus at the heart of an epidemic in one country could make it to another before its vector (the diseased individual) died, spreading diseases well beyond their previous frontiers (Bowker 1996).

To discuss these imperialistic microbes coherently across borders, classifications too had to cross boundaries, a purpose that the *ICD* undertook to satisfy. The *ICD* has never been universally accepted or consistently applied, however. Some countries, particularly tropical ones, have maintained that their concerns are inadequately represented, while others do not have the infrastructure to implement its use. The Dutch developed a double system to manage their international obligation to reporting causes of death while maintaining the decorum required by the families in relation to stigmatizing diseases. Certain causes of death would be anonymously reported to the state (syphilis, diseases of the prostate, and suicide), while more palatable causes of death were provided on the death certificate given to the families (Bowker 1996).

From its precursor documents in the 1890s, which sought to track causes of death, to its 11th revision, currently in use, each edition of the *ICD* provides a description of its scope and function, which progressively increased to include a range of new uses. In 1909, the Bertillon classification (on which the *ICD* is modeled) made clear its intent: "A statistical nomenclature of causes of death . . . has the . . . humble but practical goal of enabling statistical organizations to summarize the thousands of reports which are submitted to them in as truthful and as comparable a way as possible. Anything which would distance them from this goal should be discouraged" (Bertillon 1909, 7, translation mine). And further: "A statistical classification . . . should be . . . statistical and purely statistical" (9, translation mine). Persisting in this view, the 1957 *ICD* specifies that the purpose of a statistical classification "is primarily to furnish quantitative data that will answer questions about groups of cases" (WHO 1957, vii).

By the eighth revision of the *ICD*, however, it described new purposes, such as hospital indexing, as possible uses to be made of its classifications. The next revision expanded the functions of classification to include—beyond the statistical project—a health management role, supporting the indexing of "medical records, medical care review and ambulatory and other medical care programmes." Nonetheless, this document still distances itself from clinical classification, as "to describe the clinical picture of the patient, the codes must be more precise than those needed only for statistical groupings and trend analysis" (WHO 1977, xv).

Contemporary nosology is not contained in one text or classification document. Modern doctors and medical students are faced with an array of resources. In the past, general practitioners displayed general medical textbooks, with periodical updates, prominently on their shelves and consulted them to separate the fine crackle of acute bronchitis from the rhonchi of emphysema. Now, with the exponential expansion of medical information and improved means of information storage and display, internet-based resources have assumed a dominant role in both medical education and clinical use, pushing paper resources aside (Bove 2008). The online environment provides an immediate range of diagnoses from which to choose. Commercial electronic products such as UpToDate and Diagnosaurus provide condensed literature reviews and recommendations for diagnosis and treatment.

The diagnostic process might not employ a unique standardized classification system, but the postdiagnosis process often includes classification. Read codes, as one example, are standard for use in primary care information systems for the UK National Health Service (Swayne 1993). Devised for use in computer systems, these codes are "intended to be comprehensive, including all that health care professionals, informal carers, and patients themselves may want to say about their situation, for any purpose" (30). The read codes are used to achieve an impressive number of purposes from health data collection to public planning, marketing strategy, insurance reimbursement, treatment protocols, and practice evaluation.

By 1985, there were already more than 200 statistical systems, in the United States alone, to code health, occupational, and environmental conditions (Rothwell 1985). They include such products as the Systematized Nomenclature of Medicine, which is a coding system with a controlled vocabulary and thesaurus; the diagnosis-related groups, a classification that groups conditions on the basis of their expected resource use for fiscal purposes; and the Medical Subject Headings thesaurus, produced by the National Library of Medicine to enhance information retrieval.

The explicit goals of classification are accompanied by implicit functions as well. None are perhaps as remarkable as the degree to which classification anchors professional status within medicine and legitimizes its various branches. The ability to classify illness as true or feigned, medical or psychiatric, infectious or autoimmune distinguishes patient from doctor and establishes the authority of the medical profession. As Freidson postulates, diagnosis lends status to the doctor as they adjudicate normality and decide what counts as illness (1972, 261). Medical classifications also designate and validate the respective roles of subspecialists from within. Foucar (2001) adds that classifications "codify the interaction between contemporary sub-speciality politics and contemporary scientific classification tools" (S10). Classification has played a particularly pivotal role in defining both psychiatry's position relative to other medical specialties and dominant paradigms within the specialty.

Diagnostic and Statistical Manual of Mental Disorders

Psychiatry has always guarded the boundary between health and illness, deviance and disease (Rosenberg 2006). Those who have unusual or yet-to-be-understood physical illnesses may find their complaints explained as resulting from psychogenic causes. This tendency probably relates to the certainty that guides medicine and the difficulty that it has in gathering in behavioral or physiological outliers: a classificatory predicament. What do we do with the individual case, the idiosyncratic, the marginal or deviant that the agreed-on categories fail to accommodate? As we have seen in the preceding paragraphs, diagnosis seeks to generalize, but generalization is not always possible, and mental illness is frequently used as a residual, or "waste basket," category into which those behaviors that defy other explanations must be filed. It is not unusual for physical diseases to be incorrectly attributed to psychiatric disorder either early in the disease history of an individual or in the history of the disease itself. Multiple sclerosis and Huntington disease were both mistaken for psychosis or psychosomatic disorders (Skegg 1993; J. Stewart 1989). (See chapter 4 for more on the psychiatric explanation for medically unexplained symptoms.)

Mental illness was summarily classified in historical epidemiological texts. John Graunt (1662a) made reference to "lunaticks" and to the "sort of madman who thinks to ease themselves of their pain by leaping into hell . . . [and] die in self-murder" (21), but he did not focus on the signs of or explanations for these conditions. After all, his interest in disease was only in whether it caused death. He didn't think there was much to classify. These cases, he wrote, the "generality of the word are pretty able to distinguish" (13). He did acknowledge the chaos that was "Bedlam" (or Bethlem, an asylum run by the City of London from 1547). He could not differentiate in his accounts of causes of death those who died there as a result of their madness or from other causes (20).

There was little expansion in the classifications available for categorizing mental illness over the centuries, with only one category present in the US census of 1840. It subsumed 2 conditions: "idiocy" and "insanity." In 1880, 7 categories of mental illness became available for census takers (Gaines 1992).

By 1918, the *Statistic Manual for the Use of Institutions of the Insane* expanded these categories to 22 (Kutchins and Kirk 1997).

How mental illnesses are defined, considered, shaped, recognized, studied, and revised by medicine today is captured in the successive versions of the *DSM*. In 1952, the American Psychiatric Association (APA) published the first version of the *DSM* under the auspices of the Mental Hospital Service. This publication reflected important shifts in psychiatric practice, privileging psychodynamic and psychoanalytic approaches, acknowledging the influence of environmental factors in mental illness, and making space to consider taxonomically a range of less severe forms of mental illness treated outside of the hospital (Kutchins and Kirk 1989). It was, however, a practical document that sought to standardize nomenclature rather than define a field (Gaines 1992).

The *DSM* was a document that would be, and continues to be, revised. While the revisions are putative reflections of the advancement of medical (in this case, psychiatric) knowledge, they serve as valuable sociomedical archives for tracing beliefs, actions, power, and interests (P. Brown 1995). The first revision took place in 1968 and represented a minor exercise in categorical alignment rather than the controversial conceptual and political modification that the *DSMs* were to become. The *DSM-III* revisions were motivated by three distinct forces, according to Kirk and Kutchins (1997): public protest over the pathologization of homosexuality, clinician dissatisfaction with available disease categories (and notably the need for precision in pharmaceutical trials), and third-party payment of psychiatric care. Evidence of subspecialty politics is also clear in the *DSM-III*. Published in 1980, it exemplifies how revamping a classificatory system conveyed status and legitimacy to a languishing branch of medicine.

Psychiatry was marginalized within the medical community, its therapeutic roles assumed by nonmedical professionals, its scope of practice restricted by those who funded care. Tensions within the field and a bourgeoning antipsychiatry movement led the discipline to reconstruct psychiatric classification around symptom-based categorical diseases rather than etiologically defined entities (Mayes and Horwitz 2005). The new manual "transformed the little-used mental health manual into a biblical textbook specifically designed for scientific research, reimbursement compatibility, and by default, psychopharmacology" (263).

DSM-III also sought to site mental illness within a medical model, gaining credibility through a more scientific, biological focus. Symptoms took on a different meaning; they became signs of disease rather than symbols of distress (Gaines 1992). The histories of subsequent revisions of the *DSM* (*DSM-III-R*, *DSM-IV*, and now *DSM-5*) highlight how the *DSM* is part of an always-ongoing scientific process that makes each edition provisional and every category dynamic.

The dynamic nature of diagnoses is evidenced in the similarly dynamic title of the *DSM*. Note that the current edition is expressed as an arabic rather than a roman numeral. This is to accommodate the fluid and rapidly changing nature of diagnosis: "The rationale for this move is that it will be easier to make and indicate minor revisions in the future; thus we can anticipate that there will be *DSM-5.1*, *5.2*, and so on, before there will be major changes leading to the *DSM-6*—a much simpler process than having a *DSM-V-R* (for 'revised') or any other combinations of Roman letters and the English alphabet" (Straussner 2013).

Avoiding controversy and providing an illusion of professional consensus underpins the procedures that contribute to the *DSM* revisions. For example, the *DSM-IV* held as a working principle that no changes could be made to the previous document that did not have sound empirical foundations. As a similar criterion was not in place for the earlier version, the illusion of quality control resulted in concretizing classifications with little or no empirical grounding (Kutchins and Kirk 1997).

Kutchins and Kirk (1997) emphasize that the succeeding *DSM*s create an illusion of unified professional consensus, when in fact there is, they believe, widespread confusion, disagreement, and controversy. And yet the *DSM* still shapes the profession, and the profession in turn cements the putative professional importance of the *DSM*. Academic psychiatrists anecdotally report that reviewers for psychiatric journals request the use of *DSM* categories over any other, including the *ICD*, reinforcing its importance as the bible of psychiatry.

The *DSM*'s treatment of "homosexuality" is a poignant example both of how the *DSM* is an arbiter of diagnosis and of how controversy and political pressure shape its content. "Homosexuality" was listed in the *DSM-II* as a sexual deviation, in line with necrophilia, pedophilia, sexual sadism, and fetishism. During the early 1970s, a number of factors converged to influence its removal from the *DSM*. Kutchins and Kirk (1992, 1997) detail the various changes both in the profession and in civil rights awareness that spurred the transformation of homosexuality as a diagnostic category. I summarize their discussion here.

Kirk and Kutchins's explanation for the removal of "homosexuality" from the *DSM* relates (inversely) to the disease discovery process that Phil Brown (1995) describes as the way by which new conditions find their expression in formalized disease classification. I discuss this model in greater depth in chapter 4. In brief, this discovery process includes lay discovery, social movements, and professional and institutional factors. While laypeople or lay groups might argue that a particular set of symptoms should legitimately be considered a discrete disease entity, their ability to achieve institutional recognition is usually contingent on sympathetic doctors or institutions supporting their position.

In the case of homosexuality, a reverse process took place. What was posited as disease was actually, many argued, a variation in the range of human sexualities, and its continued promotion as diagnosable opened the door to repressive and often violent actions on the bodies, minds, and rights of gay people. Individual actions, social movements, and professional and institutional factors all came to challenge, and ultimately alter, the place of homosexuality in the *DSM*. It should be made clear that changes in the status of this diagnosis were not made on the basis of new empirical or scientific evidence but on the basis of social factors.

There were three strong forces in play at the time the *DSM-III* was being developed (Kutchins and Kirk 1997). First, gay liberation, a rights-oriented movement, had gathered momentum, particularly in light of repressive treatments used against gay men and the Stonewall riots. Second, there were changes in the way the profession was viewing its mission and place. Attempts were being made to eliminate psychoanalytic approaches from psychiatric practice, focusing less on the theoretical causation of illness and the private-practice-based discipline and more on a descriptive, research-oriented discipline that mirrored mainstream medicine. And third, Robert Spitzer, a researcher and former psychoanalyst committed to removing psychoanalytic influence from the *DSM*, believed that homosexuality could not be left diagnostically as it was in the current edition. He saw both his professional development and that of the field as being linked to a coherent diagnostic index, which required reevaluating the place of homosexuality.

It was with this context as a backdrop that gay activists staged vigorous protests against the classification of homosexuality as disease at the 1970 American Psychiatric Association conference. The Gay Psychiatric Association was created and assumed a discreet presence, and that robust debate and contestation ended in a proposal to delete homosexuality from the *DSM*, which the board of trustees of the APA voted to do in 1973 (Kutchins and Kirk 1997). The negotiation of this deletion was political, driven by polemic, values, and consensus. It was a struggle that required skilled management of opposing views.

This process of disease declassification punctuates the assemblages and boundaries that circumscribe disease and the authority to label it. It demonstrates the dynamic social character of the diagnosis and the diagnostic process. As the conversion of same-sex attraction from crime against morality to disease and then to non-disease illustrates, diagnoses are *not* prior ontological entities but *social* categories that organize, direct, explain, and sometimes control our experience of health and illness. This reinforces Bowker and Star's depiction of classifications as invisible work practices, which structure (without revealing) all of the points of view that are contained in any classification document (1999).

We are today at the *DSM-5*. It was published in 2013. This revision is still, according to Owen Whooley (2017), a tool for protecting the "bona fides" of psychiatry and promoting a biomedical vision (181). The stated intention of the fifth revision was to introduce another "paradigm shift," which it did through its introduction of "dimensionalization." This reconceived mental disorders as sitting on a continuum between normality and pathology and shifted the thinking about diagnoses away from the discrete categorization of the previous revision (and of the *ICD*) toward severity scales (Whooley 2017).

This de-categorization is possibly most publicly visible in how Asperger disorder was subsumed into autism spectrum disorder (Barker and Galardi 2015). Here, we have a collapsing of categories, which resulted in an oppositional response of an engaged lay public, upset by the disappearance of a diagnostic label that offered much more than a simple explanation. The expression to be "on the spectrum" took flight in popular culture to describe both quirky people and those with severe social debilitation. And at the same time, the "we are all on the spectrum" that dimensionalization seems to invite has been a source of dissent for those with autistic identity, as they use the distinctiveness of their condition to underpin that identity.

Revealing Classificatory Politics in Diagnosis

Zerubavel (1996) eloquently describes the social construction of difference and similarity. Once classification is established, we are inclined to think of the categories as natural, when in fact, he reminds us, nature is a continuum that is only divided into categories on the basis of our understanding and conventions. Understanding classification requires, he writes, a recognition of cognitive diversity among members of different thought communities.

Because of this, and despite its tidy and compartmentalized aims, classification of disease cannot be invariant and lawlike, nor can it ignore the social. For a condition to be classified as disease, there first must be some human recognition of its undesirability. There must also be a technical capacity to discern it and a collective will to assimilate it into the ranks of diseases rather than in, say, those of the moral, the spiritual, or the idiosyncratic. Once a particular condition is established as a disease, it must be placed within the range of diseases. Where it should sit is a decision involving, yet again, technological, social, and political factors.

The management of the nosological boundary, the splitting or grouping of conditions into "different" or "like," is not transcendent. The boundary "becomes" rather than "is" the objective organization of medical practice, and that boundary does important work. As Bowker and Star (1999) emphasize, classifications give voice to certain perspectives and silence others. The paragraphs that follow provide some examples of the selective work done by medical classification and illustrate the stakes at play.

Medicine, for example, unconsciously assigns to psychiatry temporary guardianship of boundaries between disease and health; misunderstood conditions are directed its way until their mechanisms are clarified and treatments identified (Rosenberg 2006). Conditions such as pellagra, paresis (Rosenberg 2006), multiple sclerosis (Walzl, Solomon, and Stone 2022), and other medically unexplained symptoms are shuttled to psychiatry as a catchall discipline for that which medicine does not yet understand. (I explore this in greater depth in chapter 4.)

The psychiatric diagnosis finds little favor with the lay sufferer and results in contest and conflict. Locating the unexplained in psychiatry encourages patient resistance to the stigma linked to psychosomatic disorders (Dumit 2006). While the physical explanation for a symptom confers, in most cases, a lack of personal responsibility for its onset, a psychiatric one implies that the patient might have the ability to both control and reverse the physical symptoms, an interpretation that may seem impossible to the sufferer and that brings with it stigma and shame.

Expert consensus panels commonly lead the discussions around disease classification (Aronowitz 2001), exemplifying a transition to a "big science" approach to classification (Foucar 2001), where experts appointed by authoritative bodies evaluate the evidence of the condition and make recommendations. Such an approach does not normally include a lay voice, despite the importance of lay discovery in many yet-to-be-named and often contested diseases (Callard and Perego 2021; P. Brown 2008; W. Scott 1990).

Consensus is, of course, a social process, as is membership in such panels. It, like any other social process, promotes some values and extinguishes or backgrounds others. By way of example, the "International Consensus Development Conference on Female Sexual Dysfunction," whose authoritative professional status enables its recommendations to serve as mandates, was organized by the pharmaceutical industry and supported by grants from Eli Lilly, Pentech, Pfizer, Procter & Gamble, Schering-Lough, Solway Pharmaceuticals, TAP Pharmaceuticals, and Zonagen. Its statement was produced by 19 authors who acknowledged financial or other relationships with 24 listed pharmaceutical companies (more on this in chapter 5). The findings of this committee were that urgent investigation was required to develop new classifications and definitions of sexual dysfunction (Jutel 2010a; Moynihan 2003). This paper and its findings served as the justification for numerous subsequent research reports presenting tools designed to capture this asserted reality, proposing medications to treat the conditions, and urging immediate attention to them. The interests of the experts are embedded in the classifications, which, by their design, convey the statistical potency to justify and rejustify their existence.

Clarke and Casper (1996) write about the heterogeneity of the actors involved in classification. They argue that the pap smear classification systems that have evolved and mutated over many years are evidence of a kind of boundary object. The categories themselves are not as neat as their systems would presume, and issues around what smear belongs where is far from clear cut. The old systems, the reliability of the individual laboratories, the subjective reading, and the sometimes hard-to-categorize slides compel "work-arounds" within the seemingly tidy classification system.

The boundary object, as described by Star and Griesemer (1989), is a classification that accommodates the problem of common representation in intersecting yet heterogeneous social worlds. Boundary objects have "different meanings in different social worlds but their structure is common enough to more than one world to make them recognizable, a means of translation" (393). In principle, a boundary object enables communication and acknowledges a range of interests; it is an example of negotiated order.

That the boundaries of particular classificatory boxes should meander might be seen conveniently (albeit inappropriately) as an example of the progress of science marching ever closer to the truth of conditions. The classifications of overweight and obesity are useful examples of the shifting boundaries that should be probed to understand, as Clarke and Casper (1996) propose, "what counts as biomedical knowledge, for whom, and for what purposes" (603).

Classification in medicine has long histories that are dual and yet intersecting. With numbers and generalization driving one thread and clinical advancement driving the other, they have nonetheless some commonalities and an ever-increasing tendency to substitute themselves for one another, with, notably, the statistical tradition encroaching firmly on clinical practice. This notion that numbers are more systematic than reports may underpin the drift of the *IDC* from a statistical to a clinical document. The World Health Organization website (2023b) identifies the *ICD* (today in it's 11th revision) as a tool for epidemiological, health management, and now *clinical* purposes, certainly a change from the boundaries between statistics and clinical practice set in previous revisions.

We can see one important paradox that medicine faces with regard to classification. Just as Aristotle's classification attempted to find the general in the individual, so too does medicine seek to establish similarities through classification in order to promote population health, allocate resources, focus research, and so on. Medical practice, on the contrary, focuses on the idiosyncratic individual. "The scientific basis of medicine," writes Cassell (1991), "does not recognize nor provide a methodology to deal with such individual variations on the level of patient-doctor interactions" (20). While doctors are busy classifying, patients experience their disease, and their diagnosis, in myriad ways. Patient's stories of illness are an increasingly visible part of how we understand health and disease and are published in many different forms, from memoir to vlogs and blogs, first-person documentaries, and graphic stories (Jutel 2023).

Classification is not value-free. The evidence-based practice movement (which encourages weight as a proxy measurement for activity and diet, for example) values measurement over patient report. It also marginalizes unstudied populations, such as, say, Cook Islanders or Tongans. Despite the absence of population-specific statistics, close to 70 percent of these islanders have a body mass index of $\geq$ 30 (World Obesity 2023), are identified as among the fattest populations in the world, and are not spared from the stigma associated with being "fat." (On anti-fat stigma, see Elran-Barak and Bar-Anan 2018; Lee and Pause 2016; Puhl and Heuer 2009.)

Each and every classification engages some social perspectives and shuts down others, but once a classification is established, it reproduces itself in an intuitive way that silences debate. In classifying, medicine takes a snippet of nature but often fails to recognize that the boundaries of that slice are a social consensus arrived at according to the dictates, conventions, and abilities of the field rather than already existing objects waiting to be discovered.

Hacking (2001) explains that "the idea of nature has served as a way to disguise ideology, to appear to be perfectly neutral. No study of classification can escape the obligation to examine the roots of this idea . . . no study of the word 'natural' can fail to touch on that other great ideological word, 'real'" (7). Hacking's discussion points to the fact that classification seeks a picture of an object, a "fixed target," that is true to nature. Understanding how medicine decides to see one thing as distinct from—or similar to—another can help both doctors and those who study the medical institution appreciate how medicine simultaneously approaches and distances itself from its goals of preventing suffering. It can also better reveal the uses that are made of diagnosis by nonmedical agents and how they interface (or not) with the necessary medical project of diagnostic classification.

CHAPTER TWO

Social Framing and Diagnosis

Corpulence and Fetal Death

A neighbor of mine used to encourage her daughters to eat up food they didn't like by saying, "Look at Hanan! If you don't eat up, you'll get like her." And when one of them shouted, "I like Hanan! I want to be like her," her mother said, to shut her up, "But Hanan will live all by herself. She'll never have children and nobody will ever call her Mama." How could I carry a child? Would the fetus have room, or would it be squashed up against my pelvis? How would it get its nourishment, seeing that the food I ate didn't seem to put any flesh on me?

HANAN AL-SHAYKH (1994)

Diagnosis is medicine's classification tool, and as we have seen, it must be viewed as a social product of consensus rather than a natural one. Diagnosis cannot be considered in isolation from human deliberation and agency. It is precisely the way we distinguish same from different: clustering those things that resemble one another into a group and distancing those items that don't belong is at the base of classification. That which seems to be a fact of nature in medical categorization is instead shaped by social phenomena: what we are technically able to recognize as same or different and what differences we consider to be significant. One might think that the medical diagnosis is embedded with an extra degree of realness than other categories. Doesn't the evidence-based system of medicine provide some natural proofs to underpin medical classification? There is of course a materiality to disease that, on some level, seems logically to repel social construction. Asthma, tuberculosis, and gout are all real in the sense that they have biological markers or clinical features that meet standards of evidence; you can observe them, measure them, evaluate them. Yet these features are not enough to refute the presence of a social frame for diagnosis. I am using the term "social frame" in the same way that Aronowitz (2008) does: as an alternative to "social construction," a term, he argues, that often carries confounding anti-medical and cultural relativist baggage.

Social constructionism emerged as an attempt to break with a positivist approach that considered social facts as measurable entities (P. Brown 1995). The uniform social reality of positivism was replaced by the assumption that ideas are "constructed, negotiated, reformed, fashioned and organized by human beings in their efforts to make sense of the happenings of the world" (Sarbin and Kitsuse 1994, 3). Implicit in this approach is the idea that human beings are agents, not simply passive entities or disembodied intellects that possess information (Sarbin and Kitsuse 1994).

One of the most influential foundational works in social constructionism is Peter Berger and Thomas Luckmann's *The Social Construction of Reality* (1966). Here, they argue that reality, objectivity, and facts are the product of social interactions and only appear to be external to individuals because they are sustained by the practices of many people.

Social constructionism contains four key assumptions (Burr 1995). First, it is traditionally critical of taken-for-granted knowledge. It insists that we should be highly skeptical of the idea that observations of the world "unproblematically yield its nature" (3). Knowledge is not, then, simply the reflection of some external reality. Second, social constructionism assumes that the ways we understand the world are historically and culturally specific. How we understand the world, the concepts and categories we use, are the product of our history and culture. Third, knowledge of reality is the product of everyday interactions. "Truth," and indeed "nature," as we know and describe them, are products of social processes involving negotiation between people (4). Fourth, each kind of knowledge produced through social negotiations then brings about, or invites, different kinds of action. The way we make sense of the world therefore influences what sorts of actions we engage in and how we interact with others. Following these key tenets, social constructionists argue that the proper focus of inquiry is detailed examination of the social practices.

A challenge this approach presents to the sociologist of diagnosis is that social constructionism does not adequately address the tangible physical reality of illness. Best's "contextual constructionism" provides one way out. It gives credence to the empirical world, recognizing that the human claims and categories and actions are in regard to "something" (Best 1989). The researcher should therefore also engage with this "something" to provide empirical verification to the social conditions that are being constructed. Phil Brown (1995) suggests a similar approach. He advocates for taking the physical reality seriously, while still emphasizing the importance of wider social forces and interactive decision making.

Aronowitz has skirted the issue of how disease's tangible realities are entwined with social conceptualization by avoiding the term "constructionism" completely. "Social framing," he contends, helps remove the misconception connected to social constructionism that there is no physical reality. Instead, it highlights the inevitable presence of social forces in the categories and classifications of medicine.

Social framing is the way that societies "generally recognize, define, name and categorize disease states and attribute them to a cause or a set of causes" (Aronowitz 2008, 2). But social framing also shapes the reality of those at risk of or affected by the diseases in question. In this chapter I provide two vignettes describing different medical diagnoses. Each diagnosis is, on the one hand, indisputably documentable but, on the other, is strongly framed by, or in turn frames, social as well as biological reality. I have chosen these two conditions—overweight and stillbirth—precisely because of how observable they are. Unlike diagnoses that are easy to debunk because their cultural content is so close to the surface, these are unquestionably physical realities. Although we might contest what constitutes "chronic fatigue" or argue about to what "normal" sexuality "hypoactive sexual desire disorder" is juxtaposed, we can't argue with the fact of a dead fetus. Similarly, fat can be observed, pinched, prodded, and photographed. It is hard to refute that it is there. And yet, while there is no dispute about their existence as observable phenomena, these diagnoses are also socially negotiated categories. This is why they are the perfect heuristic for highlighting social framing and its place in medical classification. And I would argue that any diagnosis, no matter how documentable, how visible, how contagious, is socially framed.

First, I consider overweight as an example of a diagnosis whose social frame is anchored in beliefs about how the body's appearance is directly linked to both its moral and physical core. I show how something as tangible as weight is still strongly associated with the social in its meaning and its presentation. Overweight is actually a new condition; it can be framed as a diagnosis only in a social context where scales are available to determine body weight (in distinction to qualitative "fatness") and where there is a prevailing confidence in the ability of statistical assessment of weight to assess individual health. I show how weight has become assimilated as a proxy measure of well-being in Western society, a practice that was initially strongly resisted and remains dubious.

Then, I talk about the fraught diagnostic terms surrounding fetal death. The implications embodied in the terms "abortion," "stillbirth," and "miscarriage" establish conflicting subject positions for the pregnant person, the parent, and the fetus and have both legal and administrative consequences for the person who failed to give birth to a live child. I have titled this chapter "corpulence and fetal death" to punctuate the fact that these conditions can be just as easily seen in nonmedical as in medical terms.

Corpulence

In 1931, Jean Leray, consultant physician at Brides-les-Bains (France) wrote a textbook titled *Embonpoint et obésité: Conceptions et thérapeutiques actuelles.* This was a book designed to present a complete technical picture of the pathology of adiposity and its remedies. Curiously, the word *embonpoint*, translated in English as "plumpness," comes from the expression *en bon point*, or "in good condition." Overweight has not always been a disease in France (or elsewhere either), as this etymology confirms.

Is it possible to think that overweight was not always perceived as a health problem? Overweight is indeed a new disease, but not because people are fatter than they once were. Rather, overweight could not exist as a category of analysis prior to the twentieth century because, while scales existed, they were too expensive for doctors' offices or for personal use. As a result, weight was not a feature of obesity. This is not to say that fatness did not exist; it featured as a topic of study in both medical and lay circles for centuries. It was mentioned, for example, by Hippocrates. Fatness and overweight, however, are two distinct concepts, and it is this distinction that provides a key to the conceptualization of overweight as a disease. The words "fat" and "obesity" are qualitative descriptions of corpulence, but neither suggests measurement or the idea of some target weight, ideal for good health. Nineteenth-century physicians viewed obesity in qualitative terms; Herrick (1889) called it an "increased bulk of the body, beyond what is sightly and healthy," and Thomas (1891) referred to it as "excessive development of the adipose tissue." Diagnosis of obesity was therefore unrelated to weight.

Today, on the contrary, obesity can be, and is, measured. The body mass index (BMI), which I discuss below, calculates corpulence by a formula comparing the weight of the body in kilograms to its height in meters squared. It's a technical, objective piece of science that doesn't require the patient to speak or the doctor to look. Weight is not only the diagnosing tool, but, when there is enough of it (and even in the absence of what could be labeled obesity), it becomes a disease in and of itself. The World Health Organization (WHO 2023a) refers to an "epidemic" of overweight. In the same way, the Centers for Disease Control and Prevention (CDC 2023) lists overweight as a "disease or condition" and links to teaching documents that explain that the prevalence of overweight has increased to "epidemic proportions." Its existence as an object of epidemiological study confirms overweight as a disease, rather than the simple descriptive adjective it used to be. Overweight and obesity are referred to in the same breath in texts of all kinds, insinuating overweight as a stepping stone to the already-well established diagnosis of obesity.

What are some possible explanations for the emergence of overweight as a disease entity? I believe that two important phenomena provide a strong foundation. The first is the importance accorded to measurement in understanding health and illness. The second is the strong emphasis that Western society places on normative appearance. These two factors are reinforced by the commercialization of self-management through the gym, diet, and pharmaceutical industries.

The Scales Don't Lie

Measurement of the body, including weight, emerged in the nineteenth century as part of a general endeavor to establish rules about humankind and of subgroups within the species. The body mass index, used today to determine overweight and obesity, was devised by Adolphe Quetelet (1870) and was motivated by the religious incentive of discovering the presence of God's rules on earth.

Body measurement was the focus of anthropometry, anthropology, phrenology, and physiognomy even before the nineteenth century. Determining character, criminality, mental illness, and racial purity on the basis of size of different body parts was a particular preoccupation of the scientific community. Lavater (1855) generated a massive catalog assigning personality traits to physical signs. Similarly, Lombroso and Ferrero (1895), in their work comparing the body types of prostitutes, female lunatics, and "normal" women wrote of measurements: "We would retain them as the frame, so to speak, of the

picture; or, rather, as the symbol, the flag of a school in whose armoury numbers furnish the most effective weapon; and we would recommend such re-
tention the more, that whenever a difference does result on measurement, the
importance of the anomaly is doubled" (2).

Using measurement for the assessment of physical health, however, was
not as prevalent. Leray, in his 1931 analysis of plumpness and obesity devotes
a number of pages to the different formulas and tables purporting to identify
the perfect healthy weight, but he reduces their importance to "theoretical
interest" and chooses rather to accept Leven's definition of safe body weight
as "[a person's] average weight, maintained over a number of years, as long as
the subject has been well" (7, translation mine). Leray argues that the correct
weight for an individual could not be determined by standardized tables. Similarly, William Christie (1927) warns readers that "no weight table is sufficient
by itself to base an estimate of the ideal state." He continues, "Standard tables
which show the average for men and women of our race at any given age and
height are fallacious, because no allowance is made for the distinctions of
personal physique, nor consideration given to obvious rolls of fat" (23).

But it did not take long before most physicians capitulated to the ease and
purported objectivity of scales in the assessment of patient health. This may
have been in part due to a change in the cost, availability, and size of scales.
At the end of the nineteenth century, the *Lancet* (1897) spoke of the presence
of scales in the doctor's consulting room, presenting the "Reliance Weighing
Machine" in its Notes and Short Comment section: "Hitherto, these personal
weighing machines have taken up too much room in a consulting room and
the expense has been too great" (1316). Later, advertisements for these scales
characterize them as "useful adjunct to the consulting room" (*Lancet* 1899,
940). Undoubtedly, as scales became more available, and as concepts of evidence in medicine were afforded more primacy, weight became an important
part of the doctor's assessment.

Hillel Schwartz (1986) argues that "the body when weighed told the truth
about the self. Once gluttony had been linked to fatness and fatness to heaviness, heaviness had still to be regularly identified by numbers on a scale, rather
than by vague and subjective sensations" (147). Doctors would be relieved to
have a straightforward mechanism for judging patient health that did not rely
upon patient reports of eating or exercise habits, or what Leray refers to above
as "wellness." The scales wouldn't lie, although the patient might. As Foucault
(1963) writes in his history of the clinic, the medical gaze saw the patient as a

barrier to the truth: "In order to know the truth of the pathological fact, the doctor must abstract the patient. . . . [T]he medical gaze . . . [addresses] all that which is visible in illness, but starting from the patient, who hides that which is visible by showing it" (8, translation mine). In the clinical assessment, the patient's story can obstruct the clinician's pursuit of the facts of the illness.

The scales for weighing a patient would become part of the trend, described by Rosenberg (2002), toward "instruments of precision" that emerged in the late nineteenth century. These apparatuses, including microscopes, thermometers, and later manometers, radiology equipment, and electrocardiogram machines, offered objective mechanisms for capturing, standardizing, and monitoring disease. Rosenberg argues that being able to express results in standardized units enabled disease to be "operationally understood and described. It was measured in units, represented in the visible forms of curves or continuous tracings" (244). This standardization and measurability form the basis of contemporary diagnosis, epidemiology, and evidence-based medicine, which produce and reproduce overweight as a disease entity.

An important tenet of evidence-based medicine is that scientific research informs clinical decisions and therapeutic approaches. Good medicine, in evidence-based practice, is when the clinician, using sound judgment and experience, artfully interprets the findings of research studies (which themselves attempt to minimize variables, bias, and researcher conflict of interest while testing for the generalizability of the findings) and applies it to the patient. But such integration is possible only in the context of standardization, where variability can be defined, populations discerned, results compared, and similarity to the patient established. Implicit therefore in the research-based or experimental model is the quantification of cause and effect—in this case, the measurement of, and focus on, body weight.

With the ability to quantify corpulence comes the potential to track its distribution, prevalence, and correlates. In turn, this allows a description of normality and a delineation of the bounds of normal build, which subsequently naturalizes concepts of difference and deviance. Numbers imply neutrality—as qualitative researchers, who have long fought for recognition of their nonquantitative methods, would report.

Yet even as scales became a standard feature of the medical rooms and a range of weight classification systems became available and was implemented, the social shaping of diagnostics options continued to vary. From 1942 to 2000, no fewer than 18 different ideal/desirable/normal/suggested/acceptable or other categorical formulations for weight were implemented by a range of official classificatory documents (Kuczmarski and Flegal 2000). A weight considered "ideal" in 1942 (say, 162 lbs. at 5'7" [73 kgs at 1m70]) would have been "desirable" in 1959, "acceptable" in 1985, and "overweight" in 2000.

Today, the current gold standard for weight assessment in the Western world is the BMI. It too, however, is a moving target. Since 1990, the upper limit of healthy weights has changed from 27.8 to 24.9, and the cut-off range for healthy weight on the basis of age and gender has been modified (Kuczmarski and Flegal 2000). Changes to the classification system are due to increasing scientific input relative to risks and benefits of particular classificatory groupings. Yet such science cannot be assumed to be either universally accepted or unproblematic. The Dietary Guidelines Advisory Committee (1995) reports that mortality increases above a BMI of 25 and recommend that this be considered the lower limit of a risk category. In contrast, Flegal and her colleagues (2005), using data from the National Health and Nutrition Examination Survey and on the basis of the estimated relative risk for mortality of BMI categories, report that overweight (< 24.9 kg/m^2) is not associated with excess mortality. Similarly, Orpana and colleagues (2009), in a study of more than 11,000 adults, find that mortality is actually *lower* in the overweight and in class 1 obesity (BMI 30–34.9).

These challenges, and others like it, to weight as a marker of wellness have not managed to unseat the scales as primary tool in the creation of the diagnosis of overweight. They continue to dictate wellness and create a convenient mechanism for understanding corpulence, one that reflects the anxiety of a society concerned with normative standards of appearance.

Normative Appearance and Health

The importance of appearance in Western culture is the second cornerstone to overweight as a medical diagnosis. While measurement underpins the creation of this condition, before it can be measured, it must occur to people that it is a concern: something that *should* be measured systematically and in the absence of complaint by the subject. We don't, for example, assess the length of the second toe as a routine part of health care, despite it being the sign and definition of Morton foot syndrome, unless the individual complains of metatarsal discomfort.

The visible presence of corpulence is pivotal in the privileging of weight as something that needs to be monitored. One's appearance, and how closely it matches normative expectations, is of great importance in Western society. Whether the standard of beauty is one of plumpness or of thinness, it is the departure from the standard that will be a source of concern embodied in social institutions, including, but not restricted to, the medical establishment, the church, and legal and educational fraternities. Not only has beauty been associated with goodness and ugliness with vice; particular forms and presentations of the human body have been associated with various meanings.

Historical attitudes toward appearance demonstrate how deviation from physical norms is problematized, condemned, and today, diagnosed. Early Christian doctrine uses metaphors of beauty to speak of virtue, with the "spotless mirror" (*speculum sine macula*) representing the goodness of the Virgin Mary and blemishes bearing witness to sin. In the fourth century Augustine described the Holy Scriptures as a mirror that reflects the truth about the self: "You're ugly, you see yourself ugly. But when you come in front of it in your ugliness and see yourself ugly, don't blame the mirror. Go back to yourself. The mirror isn't deceiving you, take care you don't deceive yourself" (1990, 336).

Throughout seventeenth- and eighteenth-century texts, appearance, particularly of a woman, was purported to reveal the inner qualities of the individual. Wealthy Renaissance families used portraits of their daughters to arrange marriages, and they were required to convey as much information as possible about the individual portrayed. Female beauty signified morality and virtue as well as membership of a particular social class. Closely linked in Renaissance thought and art, beauty and virtue were further highlighted by mottoes and emblems on the reverse of the portraits, punctuating the meaning portrayed by the primary image. The back of Leonardo da Vinci's portrait *Ginevra de' Benci* underlines the meaning of the portrait with the inscription "Beauty Adorns Virtue" (D. A. Brown 2001).

While it is not the purpose of this chapter to develop a discussion on the unequal focus of beauty as, in particular, a testimony to female virtue, it is clear that these discourses tend to target women. A highly developed notion of feminine duty is prevalent in texts from many eras and reflected in contemporary media. These texts contain strong messages about a woman's individual responsibility to achieve the normative standards of beauty.

The idea that inner character is revealed by external appearance, however, takes a different form in the nineteenth century. Virtue becomes embedded in the discourse on health maintenance. While virtue once inscribed itself on the body in the form of beauty, the new virtue is good health, which can also be discerned through an individual's appearance. In 1896, Ayer advocated its sarsaparilla as a blood cleanser: "Beauty begins in the blood" and insisted that "Beauty is blood deep, not 'skin deep'" (Ayer's Sarsaparilla 1896, 115), while the California Fig Syrup Company (1896) claimed that "one of the greatest factors in producing a clear, clean skin and therefore a perfect complexion, is the use of Syrup of Figs." And the Pabst Brewing Company (1897) lauded a young mother "flushed with perfect health" after consuming Pabst Malt Extract, the "best" tonic.

Mirroring the nineteenth-century description of health as a state of beauty, today we treat health as an aesthetic state we can assess through the shape and measurement of the body. Carole Spitzack (1990) describes health as an oppressive standard for attractiveness that heightens concerns about outward appearance. "An aesthetics of health," she states, "not only requires slenderness . . . but appropriate skin colouring, muscle conditioning, facial structure, and an absence of facial lines or 'defective' features" (36).

Art historian Barbara Stafford and ethicists John Puma and David Schiedermayer (1989) discuss the hidden role of visual and perceptual preferences in medical judgments about the abnormal. There is a standard of homogeneity, they write, that governs how medical professionals respond to patients, how the law protects patient rights, and what defines our medical priorities. Normality, the dreaded bugaboo to which we aspire in cultural practices is, not surprisingly, just as deeply ingrained in medicine. "The unstated perceptual norm that governs our reactions to patients is predicated on a symmetrical and minimalist conception of beauty. Less is more. Even wins over odd. Homogeneity is better than complexity" (214). Historically, however, physiology, ethics, and aesthetics have attempted, and continue to attempt, to capture the symmetry of beauty or of good taste in measurement and geometry. Perfection by number and by form had, and continues to have, implications for the notion of what it means to be human and what it means to be healthy, reinforcing the aesthetic of health described by Spitzack.

Being Overweight, Being Diseased?

Quite clearly, overweight is both a cultural and a medical concern in contemporary society. Vigorous gym, diet, and pharmaceutical industries pin their operations upon the anxiety of those able to pay to strive for the perfect body. Helping people to consider themselves ill or at risk of illness provides a platform for piggy-backing commercial interests onto medical authority. And creating a disease category out of a self-identifiable statistical deviation such as weight enables the commercial exploitation of those so afflicted. Self-assessment tools generate significant consumer interest (McEntee 2003). Those conditions that can easily be diagnosed by a consumer without medical intervention are particularly attractive to industry. For example, BMI calculators are popular features on weight-loss and pharmaceutical websites, such as those for the American Society for Metabolic and Bariatric Surgery or the injectable weight-loss drug Saxenda (Novo Nordisk 2023). But the weight-loss industry extends well beyond the pharmaceutical companies and plays an important role in the generation and promulgation of the diagnosis of overweight.

Many industries stand to benefit from the belief that overweight is a disease. This results in significant lobbying and product promotion based on the disease label (Oliver 2006). Weight reduction, muscle tone, and body shape are exceptionally strong markers of "health" to consumers (Spitzack 1990). The gym, diet, self-help, cosmetic, pharmaceutical, and many other industries all have a financial stake in ensuring that people see their weight as problematic from a medical point of view (Jutel and Buetow 2007).

Peter Conrad (2005) has referred to commercial interests as an important vehicle for medicalization. Examples of an implied medical endorsement for products and services are prevalent in advertising strategies, particularly in what Dixon and Banwell (2004) refer to as a "diets-making complex," or a vehicle, often exploitative, for the dominance of health considerations in all facets of dietary discourse. Transferring such information to the consumer implies recognition of lay knowledge of health risk, buttressed by authoritative medical discourse and language that draw the individual into a closed circle of virtuous consumers who focus on important evidence-based truths.

Other researchers question whether the medical concern with overweight is a dangerous case of diagnosing non-disease. Physiologist Glenn Gaesser (1999) explains that the bulk of epidemiological evidence fails to support the "lose weight–live longer paradigm" and argues that contemporary medicine disregards the protective effects of moderate overweight with respect to osteoporosis, mortality, diseases of the lungs, and some forms of cancer. A number of studies have reported that thinness and weight reduction can present a higher risk of mortality than obesity.

Gaesser points out that many independent factors covary with BMI, and teasing out those factors is a challenge. Lifestyle, exercise, and diet can affect weight and can also affect mortality and morbidity. Weight becomes a symptom rather than a cause, but nonetheless it is generally taken as a purveyor of truth in the context of evidence-based medicine. While an individual's account of activity level or dietary intake may be unreliable, BMI is purportedly free of bias. I use the word "purportedly" intentionally, for while numbers may appear free of bias, the meanings they capture are not benign. BMI is a population measurement and says nothing about the health of an individual patient. It is a measurement that does not specify the population it captures. As one example, the understudied Pacific Island populations have lower adiposity at higher BMI levels than white Europeans (Frayon et al. 2018). BMI is a crude measure of body fat and ill suited to measuring health in certain groups (Robinson et al. 2005). Recent studies have cast doubt on the validity of BMI to represent adiposity accurately and its ability to differentiate between populations (Nevill et al. 2006).

On this subject, one should note that BMI marginalizes unstudied populations, such as, for example, Cook Islanders or Niueans. Despite the absence of population-specific statistics, close to 70 percent of these islanders have BMIs of ≥ 30 (World Obesity 2023). They are identified as among the fattest populations in the word and are not spared from the stigma associated with being "fat" (on anti-fat stigma, see Elran-Barak and Bar-Anan 2018; Lee and Pause 2016; Puhl and Heuer 2009). The remoteness and small size of their populations exclude them from mainstream epidemiological study, making generalizations about the relationship between BMI and their population health unreliable.

That overweight should be a disease entity is not a surprise given the beliefs upon which Western approaches to the body are buttressed. What is salient, as Rosenberg (2002) points out, is that diagnosis poses a number of intractable social dilemmas, particularly the "difficulty inherent in fitting idiosyncratic human beings into constructed and constricting ideal-typical patterns" (251). As Cassell (1991) observes, the effect of science on clinical medicine is considerable. Science's purported neutrality, its objective generalizations about populations and about diseases, and its reduction of the human condition into physiochemical terms is at odds with clinical practice. Science is about generalization, while clinical assessment is about the individual.

The social framing of overweight as a diagnosis reflects the social reality of those who are overweight. The putative disease contains the possibility of both self-diagnosis and of self-treatment. With scales and the wide-ranging availability of diet, exercise, and over-the-counter pharmaceutical products, there are far-reaching implications for reinforcing values about normative weight and also for creating unrealistic standards and expectations that fill hapless large people with feelings of inadequacy and guilt.

Fetal Death

Just as observable and "real" as plumpness, the death of a fetus in utero is an undebatable event. It can be seen, measured, recorded, studied, and compared; however, this does not remove it from a social frame with regard to its label or to its impact. Medicine provides a range of diagnostic terms to describe death in utero: each with different consequences for the women and families affected by the event.

None of these terms is value-free; they embody a number of assumptions and beliefs about pregnancy, the mother, and the fetus. The words are part of a greater cultural and political context in which the end of any pregnancy takes place, a context that is fraught with challenges. The debates raging over whether abortion should be legal or not, and whether and when a fetus is a human being frame any unexpectedly terminated pregnancy. Does the not-yet-born-baby/fetus have an autonomous existence? While arguments may attempt to humanize the product of conception,* they often dehumanize the pregnant person. Are they, or do they provide, a hostile or nurturing "environment"? These discussions infiltrate the classifications of pregnancies that do not finish in live birth. In the upcoming pages, I explore how diagnoses of fetal death convey social values, affect social practices, and reinforce a number of conflicts that rage around pregnancy.

Giving a name or a diagnosis to a condition, or in the case of fetal death, an event, will always reflect the state of knowledge of the medical community at the time of the naming. As I have reviewed previously, that knowledge is strongly influenced by the values and concerns of the society in which the diagnosticians practice. We will see how such values infuse the diagnoses of fetal death.

The cultural content of the terms "abortion," "stillbirth," and "miscarriage" presents challenges. On the surface, these terms have simple meanings. Still-

* By referring to the "baby," I would confer, wittingly, personhood to the prenatal entity that may or may not ultimately be born. Alternatively, I could refer to the "fetus," which would suggest a nonautonomous being. Either solution is problematic in a discussion that revolves around the implications contained in language.

birth is distinguished from miscarriage and abortion by the potential viability of the fetus. Stillbirth refers to the delivery of those infants who would have been viable on the basis of gestational age at the time they left the womb but who emerged inanimate, differentiating them from the miscarried fetus/baby who could not have survived. In New Zealand, the Births, Deaths, Marriages, and Relationships Registration Act 1995 provides for the recording of information relating to births and other vital records. It defines "'still-born child' as a dead fetus that: a) weighed 400g or more when it issued from its mother; or b) issued from its mother after the 20th week of pregnancy." Other Western countries have similar definitions of stillbirth, some using both weight and gestation as defining characteristics; others using just gestation. For the purpose of establishing international comparisons, the World Health Organization (2016) recommends recording all deaths that take place in the perinatal period. This, according to the *ICD-10*, "commences at 22 completed weeks (154 days) of gestation (the time when birth weight is normally 500g), and ends seven completed days after birth."

Defining the event by gestation is not straightforward, particularly when organizations use varying gestational cutoff dates. Different countries, and even different states or regional authorities within the same countries, use a variety of parameters to label stillbirth, leading to a lack of clarity and precision in the diagnosis. Highly resourced countries generally use earlier cutoff dates than poorer ones (Lawn et al. 2009).

Stillbirth implies potential viability that was thwarted by a pathological event. Yet viability doesn't fully justify the gestational definition: what constitutes viability, like BMI, is not fixed. The state of knowledge of the medical community in a particular situation and at a particular time will determine whether it can maintain an infant born before term. This means that *when* and *where* a stillbirth takes place will determine what degree of prematurity is potentially viable. Think again of isolated island nations with limited life-support technology. Viability is thus not an absolute but is reliant on availability of resources.

This question of what gestation might reasonably reflect viability brings to mind recollections from my own nursing training in the early 1980s, when I helped look after a premature infant delivered at 28 weeks' gestation, born tragically from a mother in shock after her other children perished in a house fire. The staff looked upon the child with horror as a "failed miscarriage," and many privately shuddered, thinking about the ethics of maintaining such a premature baby. Today, of course, infants of this gestation are regularly nurtured to adulthood, testimony to advances in the ability of the medical community. Perhaps to accommodate the fact that intensive care standards change over time, and that a premature infant who is not considered to be viable today may be tomorrow, the current definition of stillbirth also includes infants who, at 21 weeks' gestation, would be unlikely to survive if born alive today. And herein resides the challenge: If some currently nonviable fetuses are included in the definition of stillbirth, why aren't others?

The paradox arises from the fact that the diagnosis assigned to the pregnancy that does not result in a live birth confers a contradictory sense of order. The families of stillborn infants, even those outside the current limits of viability, are provided ritual outlets for acknowledgment of the conception and for grief, such as certificates of birth and death, burial, and gravestone, while those of late-term miscarriages are not—despite, in many cases, feeling the loss just as acutely.

Maintaining a lower limit for the definition of stillbirth may be due in part to the legalization of voluntary abortion based upon gestational criteria. The implication of viability contained in "stillbirth" would be problematic for an aborted fetus, as it allows the rapprochement of abortion with infanticide. Underlining the ability of the fetus to live outside the womb is a prominent tool in the pro-life, anti-abortion discourse. Its ability to live autonomously is also ostensibly embodied in the miscarriage/stillbirth distinction, even in the absence of voluntary abortion. The terms themselves enforce this: "miscarriage" implies the failure of the mother/womb to protect the dependent fetus, while "stillbirth" conveys the potential of the fetus's autonomous (albeit, temporarily supported) existence and the innocence of the mother in the fetal death.*

Rosalind Petchesky (1987) argues that fetal autonomy is reinforced by the use of imaging techniques, notably in pro-life propaganda campaigns. The ultrasound image shows the baby/fetus in isolation from the pregnant person, recasting it as an autonomous subject and reducing the pregnant person, at the very most, to the passive mediator of fetal growth, "representing the fetus

---

* The term "miscarriage" simultaneously acknowledges and denies fetal personhood. On one hand, it distinguishes the child from the womb: an object to be transported, delivered, and potentially dropped. On the other, the statutory and cultural practices that accompany a miscarriage remove the autonomy of personhood upon the ending of the pregnancy, as I will discuss later. The child becomes a fetus, which is denied the trappings of death.

as primary and autonomous, the women as absent or peripheral" (268). This results in a climate where the pregnant person can be cast in an adversarial position vis-à-vis her pregnancy. According to Kathryn Conrad (2001), the pro-life movement actively promotes this position through the maintenance of fetal autonomy, identifying an array of behaviors of the pregnant person as risky and irresponsible, and positing the womb as a potentially hostile environment. The baby is depicted in its intrauterine environment, moving, breathing, and sucking its thumb. This endearing and powerful imagery emulates the family photo while erasing the woman from the frame. These images become an effective tool in the campaign to discourage voluntary abortion, as they cast the fetus as child and the invisible womb as "the most dangerous place in the world to be" (Riddick, cited in Conrad 2001, 159).

It is precisely whether the woman is attempting to give birth or, rather, to terminate the pregnancy that determines the individual meaning associated with the diagnosis assigned to the outcome of the pregnancy. The challenge to health care providers occurs when there is a mismatch between cultural and individual interpretations of where autonomy and agency reside in the birthing process. I will review the terminology used to qualify fetal death, its importance in the assessment of care, its impact on administrative processes, and the threats it may present to those who experience pregnancy loss or termination.

Naming Names

The infant mortality rate is often used as an indicator of national health. Discrepancies between nations and between different populations of the same nation are identified as major challenges to be tackled and constitute important priorities. Perinatal mortality, specifically, including stillbirth and early neonatal death, is considered the measuring tool of a maternity service's performance (Women's Health Committee 2021). This focus is undoubtedly reinforced by the symbolic importance of conception, pregnancy, and infancy in Western culture. At no other time in life is existence so dependent upon the concerted care of other human beings. At this stage in development, one can easily witness the effect of human agency on health: in the absence of intervention, survival itself is uncertain. This justifies the importance of care, and of health care in particular.

In midwifery practice, for example, stillbirth is an important measure of failure. Cultural conventions, deeply historical in origin, continually remind the midwife of the potential for the baby to perish. The modern title of the memoirs of eighteenth-century Frisian midwife Catharina Schrader is suitably extracted from a message of relief contained in her own records: "Mother and child were saved" (Schrader 1987). Contemporary conventions around the reporting of births also remind the midwife of this ominous threat. Notes by the midwife adhere to the following formula: "XX hours: spontaneous vaginal birth, *live*, female, APGARS X and Y, etc." (emphasis added). Documentation of obstetric history, birth notification, and hospital/homebirth databases contain side-by-side columns or choices for "live" or "stillborn." The New Zealand Midwifery Standards Review data sheet includes stillbirth as one measure of performance, clearly linking the professional development process of midwives to the stillbirths of babies for women under their care (New Zealand College of Midwives 2018). Stillbirth is also commonly one of the measurements of quality when comparing outcomes of total midwifery-led care and shared or obstetrician-led care, as in the famous randomized controlled trials carried out in Australia and in Sweden (Rowley et al. 1995; Waldenstrom and Turnbull 1998).

If stillbirth is a marker of professional performance, then we have to differentiate those deliveries that could never, in our contemporary setting, have resulted in a live birth (less than 21 weeks) from those that might have. The prospect of a pregnancy that could have resulted in live birth and did not strikes terror in the heart of a midwife or obstetrician. The impact of being involved in a delivery that unexpectedly does not result in live birth is horrifying. As reported by Cowan and Wainright (2001), "It does not take much to rekindle the vivid nightmares of that experience and to relive the acid adrenaline nausea of impending disaster that overwhelm [the midwife]" (313). The emotional experience of the caregiver, be they a midwife or an obstetrician, will be subordinated to the grief of the parents and will often be assaulted by litigation, marginalization, and professional scrutiny.

If, on the contrary, the delivery could never have resulted in a live birth because of the short term of the pregnancy, the consequences for the carer are different. Self-doubt and terror evaporate with the disassociation from any potential guilt. The experience of a nonviable delivery would be referred to colloquially as a "miscarriage" and would be considered unfortunate but not tragic. Within the medical community, the formal description of such an outcome is "abortion." In contrast with the popular use of this term, which signifies *deliberate* termination of pregnancy, the medical meaning simply denotes termination, with a range of adjectives to qualify it: "voluntary," "incomplete," "spontaneous," "threatened," "legal," "illegal," or "recurrent." Curiously, the legal definition of abortion is quite different from the medical one. While the etymology is from the Latin *aboriri*, "to miscarry" (*ab*, "away from," plus *oriri*, "to be born"), in New Zealand, the Crimes Act 1961 defines abortion in terms of intentionality: the "procurement of miscarriage," in line with, and reinforcing, lay definitions of the term—signifying intention on the part of the parturient and lending to confusion as a result of the liability inherent in the term.

Whether a death is a miscarriage, a stillbirth, or an abortion will have not only legal but also fiscal and cultural implications. As Wilfred Mills (1977) pointed out in the *Lancet* many years ago, the distinction between an abortion and a neonatal death has non-negligible social consequences: "A neonatal death will carry a birth and death certificate and thus an entitlement to a financial maternity benefit that would be lost if the event were classed as a late abortion."* This holds true today. Work and Income, the source of welfare support in New Zealand, will award a funeral grant only for infants who were either born live or who fit the statutory definition of stillborn (HealthEd 2022).

Similarly, the New Zealand Births, Deaths, Marriages, and Relationships Registration Act does not accord personhood when there is a miscarriage as opposed to a stillbirth. According to the interpretation of the act, "child" includes a stillborn child, while "miscarriage" refers to the "issue from its mother . . . of a dead fetus." While the bearer of either is considered a mother, she is entitled to refer to her "child" only if it meets a statutory requirement of 21 weeks' gestation or 400 grams weight.

This statutory principle presents challenges. Midwives recall the difficulties encountered less than two decades ago if a multiple birth took place before the then-statutory definition of viability at 28 weeks. One twin might not survive birth, while another might live but die later. The existence of the twin who did not survive birth is not acknowledged in the same way as that of the one who did: the stillborn baby cannot be registered. Breathing outside the womb, rather than gestation, conferred the status of child. With the renewed definition of stillbirth resting upon 21 weeks' gestation, one might presume that this problem is resolved, but with the technical advances in neonatal in-

---

*   Here, the medical sense of early death, rather than criminal procurement, is implied by the word "abortion."

tensive care, babies are resuscitated and saved at increasingly early gestational stages.

Not all peoples use viability or gestation in their assessment of personhood. The Indigenous people of New Zealand, the Māori, have a different perspective on pre-birth. Māori practices do not use gestational age as a distinguishing category, calling the pre-born child *pepi*—the same name used for a child after its birth—regardless of its developmental stage. The *pepi* also has agency and decides to inhabit or to leave the womb. The cultural approach to the death of the *pepi* would not be affected by its gestational age either but would be constrained nonetheless by New Zealand statutory definitions. A *pepi* not considered a child by the Births, Deaths, Marriages, and Relationships Registration Act, because of early gestational age, could be buried on the *urupā*, the traditional Māori burial place (Khyla Russell, pers. comm. 2005), but in no other cemetery. Death before breathing is a prominent feature of Polynesian stories of creation, with Maui, the iconic Māori demigod hero, having left his mother's womb *pepi mate*, or stillborn, to be rescued by Tangaroa (god of the seas) and raised by Tamanuikiterangi (Erlbeck 2001).

In European culture, by contrast, the difference between stillbirth and miscarriage brought, and continues to bring, other legal consequences beyond death registration and legal burial. Unmarried women who lost their babies were subject to suspicion that they might have killed the baby to avoid the infamy of bringing an illegitimate child into the world. While a miscarriage was unfortunate, a stillbirth cast suspicion. European women suspected of infanticide in the eighteenth century described their miscarriage as the delivery of "only blood" or of a substance "like a lump of flesh," thus denying the existence of a baby and placing the event in the realm of a "false conception" rather than a birth marred by infant death (M. Jackson 1996). One might see parallels here with the recent case of "Baby Aaron," the much reported discovery of a stillborn child in the sewage system of Hastings, New Zealand (One News 2005).

While there was no doubt, according to the coroner's report, that the child was born dead, the mother still risked charges and prosecution. Disposing of a dead baby is a violation of section 181 of the Crimes Act, which states that "everyone is liable to imprisonment for a term not exceeding 2 years who disposes of the dead body of any child in any manner with intent to conceal the fact of its birth, whether the child died before, or during, or after birth" (NZ Parliamentary Counsel Office 1961). The act does not define what constitutes a child, but it is clear that how the term is used is of fundamental importance. If the event constituted a stillbirth, the woman may be charged with a crime, while if it were a miscarriage, she would not be called to account.

Since "Baby Aaron" was discovered to be the fetus of a young unmarried teen (One News 2005), one could speculate that its flushing away was evidence of the girl's denial of its personhood and also perhaps an attempt to preserve her own reputation. In this case, the construction of the event as birth or non-birth and the fetus as child or non-child has far-reaching legal and personal consequences.

While some continuity in practices surrounding the early termination of pregnancy might be present, representations of miscarriage vary according to the era in which it occurs. Leslie Reagan (2003) argues that today's pregnancy-loss movement draws on both the current anti-abortion and feminist movements to comprehend and define miscarriage, female emotion, and motherhood. She also maintains that attitudes toward miscarriage have changed. In the twentieth century, miscarriage has variably been seen as a hazard, a blessing, or a tragedy, depending on its place in time.

The challenge presented by the issues surrounding a pregnancy that does not result in a live birth results in the paradox of conflicting maternal subjectivities. On the one hand, articulating fetal personhood simultaneously conveys to the mother the burden of guilt and the responsibility of care (depending upon the birth outcome and the mother's participation in its achievement). This feto-centric model of pregnancy may also result in the removal of maternal subjectivity. On the other hand, denying fetal personhood denies maternity by creating the childless mother. Importantly, the values embodied in the terminology used in New Zealand texts can be at odds with the experiences of individual women. Petchesky (1987) points out a similar mismatch in women's views of fetal ultrasound images. Although the woman would seemingly be disempowered by removing her from the picture, thus treating her as a maternal environment without agency, pregnant people do not necessarily experience these images negatively. The response is always contingent upon individual circumstances—mainly on whether the person wishes to be pregnant. For one woman, these images are an unproblematic first peek at a soon-to-emerge baby, for another, they are an instrument of intimidation, creating a female subject, otherwise effaced by medical imaging technology, who is morally deficient and dangerous.

Likewise, the manner in which fetal death is received by pregnant people, their partners, families, support systems, and health professionals depends upon complex individual social and psychological circumstances. While one group might experience gestational death as loss, another might see it as relief—and indeed could voluntarily provoke it. The subject positions available to any woman who has experienced the gestational death of her child are what is problematic. And yet, the individuals do not have the ability to change the diagnoses, the statutes, the laws, and the welfare benefits that reinforce these awkward positions. The value content of the language cannot simply be eradicated or modified to suit the circumstance, and the impact of the diagnostic category on death benefits, legal responsibility, and social recognition are considerable.

Health care professionals working within the context of pregnancies that do not result in the birth of a live infant cannot ignore the values contained in the diagnosis, particularly the conflicting potential impact on the parents who have experienced this event as a "death" in the womb. At one level, it's quite obvious: despite the innocuousness of the term in the medical community, a midwife, nurse, or obstetrician would carefully avoid making reference to "spontaneous abortion" in the face of a grieving parent who had wanted to carry their infant to term. The connotation of this word in the lay population is simply too powerful to be ignored.

Frame and Be Framed

The very real conditions of corpulence and fetal death take root as they become actualized as medical diagnoses. The authority of medicine gives substance to their existence in different ways than if they remained outside its jurisdiction. The doctor rules on the fetal gestation, acting as a catalyst for legal, economic, and social events.

With respect to fetal death, medicine's authority first to pronounce what constitutes viability in gestational terms and second to reckon the gestation is contingent on cultural and technological factors. The same holds true for corpulence. As we look at current medically sanctioned ideal weights, we see contradictions that are somehow trumped by medical positions that seem to be based in something other than science.

Paul Campos and his colleagues (2006) doubt that the putative obesity epidemic is the public health crisis it is cast to be by public health authorities and the media. They refute the assertion that there is evidence of an epidemic at all. The changes in population weight are subtle with a slight trend upward, hardly evidence of dramatic change in population health. Further, the increasing rates of BMI are not contributing to increased risk of mortality; general life expectancy continued to increase (until 2020 and the advent of COVID-19 [CDC 2022]), with the lowest morbidity and mortality in so-called overweight categories. Statistical linkages between overweight and mortality are flawed, with inadequate control of factors such as exercise, diet, and demographics. Cardiovascular risk factors have also dropped in all weight categories (Flegal 2006). What justifies this focus on obesity if the epidemiology doesn't support the argument?

Campos and colleagues (2006) posit that this is a moral panic rather than a health crisis. Moral panics are "typical during times of rapid social change and involve an exaggeration or fabrication of risks, the use of disaster analogies, and the projection of societal anxieties onto a stigmatized group or an episode" (58). Cast by the mass media as a threat to social values and interests, the moral panic is supported by "right thinking people," monitored and validated by socially accredited experts (M. Cohen 1980, 9). Moral panics have been triggered by other social phenomena, such as drug taking, crime waves, terrorism, and now, perhaps, overweight.

Considering how the proposed obesity epidemic fits the criteria of a moral panic, it helps to critique the classification of overweight as a disease. While use of the word "epidemic" may be only metaphorical, it conveys an urgency previously reserved for the plague, tuberculosis, or other major infectious events. In the traditional epidemic, rapid containment is vital to the survival, or at least the well-being, of the community. With events such as the gradual rise in population BMI, the threat takes an extremely different form. The clichéd use of the word "epidemic" is linked to specific rhetorical and policy goals and has dramaturgic aims (Rosenberg 1992). "The intent is clear enough: to clothe certain undesirable yet blandly tolerated social phenomena in the emotional urgency associated with a 'real' epidemic" (280).

In the case of the obesity epidemic, the language used is one of exigency. Obesity is seen as a threat to be fought, an insidious danger. The urgency of this message and the reasons for which a language of epidemic and doom are proposed to describe the problems of obesity forces us to consider the question of deviance. Deviance, in all cases, is attributed rather than inherent (Conrad and Schneider 1980). It can exist only in the presence of a grouping of subjects. That is to say one can be deviant only in relation *to* someone or *from* something else. Being corpulent in isolation is not deviant and indeed is, or has been, normative in some settings and eras.

There are a range of definitional questions which should be asked by a student of deviance: "Why does a particular rule, the infraction of which constitutes deviance, exist at all? What are the processes and procedures involved in identifying someone as a deviant and applying the rule to [them]? What are the effects and consequences of this application, both for society and the individual?" (M. Cohen 1980, 13).

The rules in the case of obesity, and in its definition as deviant, are shaped by overlapping and conflicting fiscal interests. I've spoken about the financial gains to be made in the promotion, control, regulation, and treatment of obesity. But the interests may be other than financial. The CDC, for example, uses the threat of the obesity epidemic as an arm in the battle for increased funding for their policy initiatives and authority (Campos et al. 2006).

Diagnoses do capture reality, but that reality is fluid, situated, and social. Mirowsky and Ross (1989) have compared diagnoses to constellations in the sky, composed of stars that are truly present but whose meaning comes from how we assemble them in recognizable patterns. The process by which a diagnosis emerges involves human—and by extension, social—discernment with all its accompanying baggage: technological, political, and cultural. A collective cultural position determines which symptoms we will see, which we will brush off as insignificant, how we make sense of what is there, and what social consequences the diagnosis will convey.

One mistaken response to the sociology of diagnosis is that it is a way of understanding a particular kind of diagnosis: the diagnosis that is psychiatric, linked to social behavior, or otherwise contested (as the next chapter will explore). But to believe this would be to limit the scope of the important sociologic consideration of diagnosis. Since the publication of the first edition of this book and notably, since the start of the COVID-19 pandemic, I have tasked myself with applying the social model to all forms of material illness. They are no less amenable to this analysis. I demonstrate this again in chapter 7, the COVID-19 chapter, where we can see how material conditions transformed into diagnoses have rich social content, as much as any other diagnosis.

Returning to corpulence and fetal death, in both, the lay perspective may be at odds with or disregarded by the medical diagnosis. Classification of overweight does not consider diet, exercise patterns, or even adiposity. Similarly, the "spontaneous first-term abortion" does not capture the feelings a pregnant person experiences at what she may consider to be the death of her child. Hunter describes how the lay and medical explanations can be at odds: the "transformed and medicalised narrative may be alien to the patient: strange depersonalized, unlived and unlivable. Returned to the patient in this alien form the medical narrative is all but unrecognizable as a version of the patient's story—and all but useless as an explanation of the patient's experience" (Hunter 1991, 13). The medical diagnosis does not consider how the individual has actually lived, explained and accounted for their condition, and cannot necessarily be incorporated into their personal narrative.

This medical-lay discordance is at the base of the next chapter, which explores how diagnosis sits at the heart of the lay-professional encounter, as a justification for consultation and a source of potential collaboration: cure but also contest.

CHAPTER THREE

What's Wrong with Me?

Diagnosis and the Patient-Doctor Relationship

> I jumped up and shook hands with this man who'd just given me
> something no one else on earth had ever given me
> I may have even thanked him habit being so strong
> RAYMOND CARVER (1998)

Hippocrates wrote that "if [the doctor] is able to tell his patients when he [*sic*] visits them not only about their past and present symptoms, but also to tell them what is going to happen, as well as to fill in the details they have omitted, he will increase his reputation as a medical practitioner and people will have no qualms in putting themselves under his care" (1983, 170). His words underline that diagnosis is at the heart of both confirming the professional status of the doctor and delineating the doctor-patient relationship, providing a rationale for the consultation, confirming the authority and prestige of the medical profession, and delegating the responsibility for labeling an illness.

Raymond Carver's poignant, autobiographical poem describes him receiving a life-threatening diagnosis. But it underscores how his own emotions and those of the doctor overlap and feed off each other, as he effaces himself before the doctor. Both submissive and generous, he holds back on causing unnecessary distress by reflecting his own pain back on the doctor while he endures this life-altering moment. Despite Carver's concern for the doctor's feelings, the doctor and patient sit in different positions in this encounter—framed by diagnosis—while nonetheless sharing its impact. The differences are grounded in perspective, education, experience, identity, emotion, and more. In this chapter, I explore some of these differences and their consequences. I begin with the illness/disease dichotomy, which describes how the matter of "not feeling well" becomes part of a medical narrative with diagnosis at its core. Then we see how the authority afforded medicine grants it the right to determine the narrative of illness and its subsequent management. Finally, I discuss the changing roles of layperson and health professional in the diagnostic encounter and envision the potential this has for the study of health and illness identities in the twenty-first century.

Illness and Disease

The pursuit of diagnosis brings patient and doctor together. Feeling unwell is the usual prompt for seeking medical attention. And it involves a premedical assessment in which the individual attributes their unwellness to what they think is likely to be a disease rather than an external or nonmedical factor. But it is the inability of the layperson to fully interpret the situation, despite assigning it to the realm of the medical, that leads to the clinical encounter (Leder 1990). The person seeks the explanatory power of the diagnosis, which the doctor is authorized to deliver.

The layperson's desire to understand their discomfort—the cough, the rash, the swelling, or the cramp—prompts this encounter with their doctor. The process by which the illness is conveyed in the consultation, in which the complaint is described and contextualized, is the first step in "organizing" an illness (Balint 1964). Balint's model of patient-doctor interaction sees the patient's pursuit of medical opinion as an organizational task. This model remains relevant to contemporary lay-professional relations. Indeed, it may have even more pertinence in the era of the increasing patient autonomy and knowledge. The patient consults the doctor to present an organizing explanation of their ailments for confirmation. In a sense, they "propose" a diagnosis.

Balint puts great emphasis on the diagnosis. The most pressing and immediate problem for the patient is "*the request for the name of the illness, for a diagnosis. It is only [then] that the patient asks for therapy*" (1964, 25). The illness proposal must be recognized by and negotiated with the doctor. This interaction might take the form of a presentation of symptoms. Already, the first step in organization has taken place. "I have a headache. Do you think it might be a tumor?" enables the doctor to organize the information gathering. Why do you think it might be a tumor? What is the nature of the pain? Have you any changes in your visual fields? The doctor ideally proceeds to a sequence of steps that rule in or out (in order of seriousness) the possible explanatory diagnoses, from brain tumor to migraine, stress, or benign headache. In the ideal encounter, or series of encounters, the doctor responds to the illness as offered, exploring the patient's organizational strategy, testing its pathophysiological coherence, offering alternative diagnoses until both patient and doctor can agree on the fundamental diagnosis underpinning the patient complaint.

Diagnosis is the medical reading of these symptoms: interpreting and organizing them according to models and patterns recognized by the profession. Leder (1990) describes this process as a "clinical hermeneutic" or interpretive project. The individual initiates an encounter with the doctor to obtain an explanatory position from which to approach the illness.

The distinction between illness and disease is important to the sociology of diagnosis. This differentiation was not made clear in earlier sociological texts. Freidson (1972), for example, used the terms interchangeably. Today, however, the distinction contains important conceptual differences that inform discussions of diagnosis. Illness is the personal experience of sickness (Kleinman, Eisenberg, and Good 1978). Illness problems are those that result from undesirable changes in social or personal function. How an individual perceives these problems, explains or labels them, and seeks remedy originates from a cultural context. This in turn influences the decision to access, or the response to, medical services. In any case, as Locker (1981) points out, to consider oneself ill is to presume a biological cause for a disvalued state of being.

Disease, in contrast, is framed by the biological rather than the personal. This is not to say that it is bereft of cultural content; rather, it represents what Western medicine considers biological or psychophysiological dysfunction (Kleinman, Eisenberg, and Good 1978). Fleischman (1999) refers to diseases as conceptual entities, or "categories of clinical taxonomy . . . extrapolated from an aggregate of similar illnesses on the basis of what is thought to be common to the illnesses so classified" (7). Disease is diagnosed, illness is not; rather, it is presented to a clinician as *presumed* disease. The transformation from illness to disease takes place through the intermediary of the doctor and the diagnosis.

While not all illnesses can be diagnosed, their narratives are the starting point for diagnosis. Note that there is more than one narrative: the patient's and the doctor's stories juxtapose and merge for a diagnosis to materialize. Patient stories, emerging from their own experience, culture, and consideration of the role of the doctor, are transformed into medical accounts upon their telling. The doctor interrogates, interprets, and retells the story, establishing the "plot" and a diagnostic organization (Hunter 1991). In Leder's model, the patient has already determined that the explanation for their discomfort is medical and that it is a doctor (rather than a different social authority, say, a rabbi or a lawyer) who will confer meaning on the narrative. Illness is the story that results when an individual sees the interpretation in terms of health and medicine. In contrast, diagnosis is the story of medicine, told in the language of disease. "In the narrow biological terms of the biomedical model," says Kleinman (1988), "this means that disease is reconfigured *only* as an alteration in biological structure or functioning" (5–6).

Arthur Frank (1995) claims that a social expectation of being ill is not just seeking care but "a *narrative surrender*" in which the patient's story is relinquished to the doctor's, which is told through diagnosis and is "the one against which others are ultimately judged true or false, useful or not" (5–6). Kleinman maintains that doctors are taught to be skeptical of patients' narratives about illness, a view shared by Foucault (1963), who writes that clinical medicine sought unequivocally to silence the patient, "who, . . . by trying to show things, ends up concealing them" (8, translation mine).

The diagnosis thus confers legitimacy to illness yet does not necessarily align with the patient's narrative for a number of reasons, not least of which is the position from which the stories are recounted. Illness narratives "reveal what life is like for the narrator . . . [including] the practical consequences of managing symptoms, reduced mobility and so on. In telling their story, individuals also reveal, or indeed may assert, their self and social identity" (Nettleton et al. 2004, 49). Medical narratives come from an institutional position, which presumes the absence of the lived experience. It is the objectivity of scientific classification (in this case, the diagnosis) that confers authority to the label. Diagnosis is the fulcrum of the medical narrative. The judgment that this implies, as Frank asserts, may deny the self and social identity that the story of illness embodies.

Frank refers to illness as the experience of living through disease. It begins, he writes, "when popular experience is overtaken by technical expertise, including complex organizations of treatment. Folk no longer go to bed and die, cared for by family members. . . . [They] go to paid professionals who reinterpret their pains as symptoms, using a specialized language that is unfamiliar and overwhelming" (1995, 5).

The languages of disease and illness may be peculiarly discordant. "A transformed and medicalized narrative may be alien to the patient: strange, depersonalized, unlived and unlivable. Returned to the patient in this alien form the medical narrative is all but unrecognizable as a version of the patient's story—and all but useless as an explanation of the patient's experience" (Hunter 1991, 13). Such alienation occurs when the medical model takes inadequate account of the illness problems (such as how the patient has actually lived, explained, and accounted for their dysfunction) and is unable to incorporate this in its own narrative via the diagnostic label.

Blaxter (2009) movingly describes her personal trajectory of illness and the means by which the process of diagnosis effaced her lived experience of disease. Diagnostic technology replaced her own voice as the focus of medical attention. Symptoms and patient history were subordinated to scan results; patient knowledge and information, even clinical examination, took a backseat. In Blaxter's experience, the abnormal PET scan result could be explained as a "shadow" from her youth, possibly a vestige of a childhood tuberculosis—an explanation refuted rather hastily by her lung specialist.

The degree to which personal and professional narratives align may contribute to health outcomes. How these narratives are enabled, heard, and exchanged makes a big difference in the framing of the diagnosis. The medical authority is salient here. Enabling a patient story—its plot, characters, setting, and description (rather than inserting the patient's words into a clinical picture)—acknowledges the patient's expertise in the construction of illness. It allows "joint authorship" by doctor and patient of the explanatory framework, the therapeutic decision, and the clinical outcomes (Clark and Mishler 1992).

Medical Authority

Diagnoses and their classificatory systems are an important collective arrangement that defines and enables the influence of professional medicine. But at an individual level, diagnosing confers power to the doctor as allocator of resources (de Swaan 1989). The diagnosis legitimizes sickness. As discussed previously, when a doctor deems a patient's condition to be medical, the latter receives previously unauthorized privileges such as permission to be absent from work, priority parking, insurance benefits, reimbursement for treatment, or access to services. The doctor certifies the complaint as "real," and "medical advice" informs administrative and policy decisions.

Authority in medicine comes from its ability to define and delineate behaviors, persons, and conditions, write Peter Conrad and Joseph Schneider (1980), but also from the organization and structure of the medical profession. Medicine has an officially approved monopoly over the right to define health and to treat illness, which results in its high public esteem. The doctor, as the agent of medicine, is accorded a prominent position in the hierarchy of expertise and a mandate to exercise their authority over that of other health professionals and laypeople (Freidson 1972).

The medical dominance articulated by Freidson is not, however, immutable. In 1988, Light and Levine argued that the power of the medical profession was already in decline, as evidenced by the introduction of malpractice lawsuits, profit-driven administration of physician performance, and cost-management strategies in medicine. More recent evidence of change in the status of doctors is present in increasing patient complaints, increasing use of alternative therapies, critical media portrayals of doctors, and lack of financial autonomy. Further, wider access to information has led to changes in the doctor-patient relationship, with patients more willing to challenge their doctor, dispute findings, or seek advice outside of the doctor-patient relationship (Heritage and Maynard 2006). Doctors are not alone today in the authority to diagnose. A range of other professionals, including chiropractors, nurse practitioners, and physiotherapists, may diagnose certain conditions in some countries.

The patient-doctor relationship was historically one of an authoritative, paternalistic manager of care with a submissive, patient* recipient. In 1939, G. Canby Robinson described the relation of doctor and patient as unique: "The natural authority of the doctor, the confidence the patient feels in his professional knowledge, his unselfish, disinterested respect for intimate communications, the tradition, so long accepted, that the relationship between doctor and patient is confidential and the sentiment of the patient that the more the doctor knows about him, the more helpful he can be, all these attitudes and assumptions establish a basis for free and unbiased communication that is possible in few other human situations" (2).

This relationship resulted, in part, from an imbalance in knowledge. The

---

* The adjective "patient" is used consciously, with an awareness of the overlapping significance of its nominal and adjectival forms.

circulation of information about pathophysiology and normal biophysical function was limited to particular professional and scientific circles. In 1958, for example, Pratt, Seligmann, and Reader noted low levels of patient participation in doctor-patient interactions. They attributed this to patients having limited understanding of their diseases and their etiologies and treatments. Patients neither expected nor requested information from their physicians. In turn, physicians acknowledged their ignorance, viewing it as a liability in terms of patient compliance, or likelihood they will accept and follow the doctor's interpretation, explanation, and recommended treatment of disease. It is a paternalistic interaction, where the patient is like a child, submitting to the guardianship of a kind and compassionate physician (Emanuel and Emanuel 1992). Patient autonomy is contained in assent and is subordinate to the beneficence of the physician.

Changing Roles in Diagnosis

Yet recently there have been assaults on the diagnostic role of medicine coming from all angles. Lay social movements advocate for diagnosis and recognition of conditions often refuted by the medical institution (Brown and Zavestoski 2004). Avid commercial forces have been eager to tap the modern patient's increased access to previously privileged medical information, seeing in self-diagnosis an excellent avenue by which to promote particular conditions and, by extension, their concordant therapies (Healy 2006). But health policies too have encouraged a transformation of traditional relationships in health care, emphasizing a more active role for the layperson, whose expertise is derived from experience rather than knowledge (Wilson 2001).

Seeking other avenues for diagnosis is not a new phenomenon, for, just as Hippocrates described the importance of the medical diagnosis, so too did he describe the unruly patient, reluctant to submit to medical care. He questioned their resolve: "Although they have no wish to die, they have not the courage to be patient." He wrote, "Is it not more likely that they will disobey their doctors rather than that the doctors . . . will prescribe the wrong remedies?" (Hippocrates 1983, 142). He emphasized the knowledge gap between layperson and doctor: "The symptoms which patients with internal diseases describe to their physicians are based on guesses about a possible cause rather than knowledge about it. If they knew what caused their sickness, they would know how to prevent it" (145).

Today, however, laypeople are far more likely to have specialized information about what causes their illness than in Hippocrates's time. Clinical decision making has changed its locus, according to Nettleton (2004). The layperson who consults the health care professional is no longer the submissive and compliant "patient" but an expert partner who brings their experience of illness to the differentially specialized medical practitioner. Medical knowledge has escaped ("e-scaped," in Nettleton's phrase), flowing as information through myriad electronic networks and internet sources, enabling the patient to access and interpret information about disease well before their encounter with the doctor.

The Health Information National Trends Survey asked respondents their first source of information when they had a question about their health: 70.1 percent would go to the internet first, with only 17.2 percent starting with their doctor or health care provider. In 2008, the numbers were 58.1 percent and 14.7 percent, respectively.

The power of the physician may be diluted by the availability of medical knowledge outside of the halls of learning. This is both because there may be a range of simple problems a person can now look after themselves but also because the patient comes to the encounter "informed," albeit sometimes "misinformed," rather than as acquiescent. They enter the clinical encounter with a different agenda than in the situation described by Pratt and colleagues (1958). The relationship is not quite as much a one-way power dependency as an encounter based on shared (albeit unequal) knowledge about health and disease.

We should not, however, be lured into thinking that during the pre-internet era the submissive patient was completely dependent on the authoritative clinician, an archetypal professional relationship. Anxiety about the proliferation and use of medical information by laypeople has troubled doctors for more than a century. In 1898, Robert Gersuny, in his hints to doctors and patients, wrote, "Sick people who . . . have read up their complaint in some book, are a great source of trouble to their doctors and themselves" (29), just as doctors of the twentieth century fretted over something akin to today's cyberphobia. Surgeon Albert Krecke explained that the patient "has heard so much about all manner of diseases that every time he feels a little poorly, he imagines the worst" (1934, 35).

Like today's clinicians, our medical predecessors lamented inadequate lay understanding of disease. The layperson is ignorant and emotional, according to the vice president of the British Medical Association, Henry Brackenbury (1934): "The lay mind, even if what is commonly regarded as well educated, is unable to form any sort of clear image of anatomical or pathological conditions. . . . [C]ommon use of medical terms and glib talk about illness, which seems to indicate that the layman is hardly aware of his own ignorance" (206). But such ignorance didn't prevent self-diagnosis, and R. F. Lapham warned that "the physician must ever be on his guard lest he unconsciously follow along the line of reasoning of the patient, or allow himself to be prejudiced or influenced by the diagnosis given by the patient" (1937, 23).

Many comments from nineteenth- and early twentieth-century doctors sound more than vaguely familiar to today's physicians. The heart of the problem may not lie in the availability of, and use by laypeople, of medicalized information, because, as history attests, this has been the case for decades. Yes, industry has perhaps a wider reach now and more tools at its disposal for communicating its messages. And the public may be more uniformly schooled, or at least equipped, in the use of the media that distribute these commercial messages. But it is important to consider that for self-diagnosis to maintain its hold, we have to consider why diagnosis matters to the patient. It is facile to reply that it is the link with treatment and prognosis that makes diagnosis important. Of course. But that is not all. Diagnosis fulfills many other social functions, as the previous chapters have underlined.

As Crenner notes in his history of Richard Cabot's early nineteenth-century private diagnostic practice (2005), even while diagnosis was fundamental to the power of the medical profession, Cabot's patients tried to use the same technical language of diagnosis that he did in their correspondence with him. With their carefully cultivated belief in the power of scientific medicine, they provided what they believed were clues to the mystery of diagnosis.

Faith in diagnosis as a means of understanding dysfunction is thus pivotal simultaneously to the expansion of medicine's reach and also to the cultivation of self-diagnosing patients. One the one hand, medicine asks patients to believe in diagnosis as an explanatory framework. On the other, doctors are dismayed that they should use diagnosis to explain what ails them. It's a conundrum.

We might turn to the past for some words of wisdom about lay access to medical information, which seemingly went against the flow. In 1936, the oncologist Frank Rector believed in the power of medical information and advocated its liberal distribution to patients. He complained that too many physicians treated cancer patients as if they were neurotic and needed to be protected from information about their disease. He countered that giving patients information allowed them to cooperate and participate fully in their care.

Many contemporary doctors incorporate the information that their patients bring with them to the consultation as part of their patient history. It helps the doctors to understand more about patients themselves and the nature of their worries. It also provides a teaching moment, where the physician can help the patient to navigate sources of information about what ails them. The words that Rector used in 1936 are good food for thought for today's clinicians. "With the new information that is accumulating daily and with the intelligent lay interest," he wrote, "the outlook is bright" (5).

Transforming the place of medical authority is not without challenges. Positioning patients as consumers opens the door for them to become the vulnerable prey of disease mongers. Indeed, the ability to assess the quality, reliability, and morality of health information is not necessarily within the grasp of most laypeople, presenting a difficulty on two fronts. On one hand, any attempt to mediate access to information or to recapture control of its delivery will infringe on lay autonomy, returning the patient to the paternalistic care of the omniscient physician. On the other, consuming information without adequate understanding puts the patient, the doctor, and the doctor-patient relationship at risk. This is most evident in self-diagnosis, which can overturn traditional diagnostic responsibilities.

Self-diagnosis serves as an important tool in public health, or at least self-prediagnosis does. Whether it's influenza or COVID-19, public health initiatives seek to reduce the spread by either asking people to stay home (as opposed to "go see the doctor") if they have "the flu." With COVID-19, of course, we advise self-isolation and rapid antigen testing. The principle, for the diagnosis scholar, is to see how self-isolation links to self-*diagnosis*.

Self-diagnosis is also widely promoted by disease-awareness campaigns, encouraging individuals to self-identify with a particular disorder and bypass the conventional diagnostic processes. It may be to bring awareness to a particular condition to promote its remedy, prompting the individual to recognize signs of the disorder, present them to the doctor, and ask whether "[name of remedy] is right for you." Or it may be to encourage early awareness of conditions for which the outcome is more favorable when detected early. Both forms of self-diagnosis present challenges to medicine as they redefine roles in the doctor-patient relationship.

If we were to ask doctors about their views, they'd likely say that patient safety is why they oppose patient involvement in diagnosis. The patient has inadequate training to consider differential diagnoses and would likely overlook other morbidities. They would argue that inaccurate diagnosis leads to delays in the treatment of more serious disorders. But, for many conditions, the doctor no longer need gatekeep treatment. For example, in many countries, medication to treat fungal infection is readily available without prescription.

The first approval for an over-the-counter (OTC) antifungal was made in the United States in 1990. Many other countries followed suit. This approval led to a reduction in prescription costs and physician services (Gurwitz, McLaughlin, and Fish 1995) but an increase in pharmaceutical sales (Ferris, Dekle, and Litaker 1996). The result of the switch from prescription to OTC medication likely contributed to a shift of financial burden from the insurer to the health consumer (Harrington and Shepherd 2002).

Accompanying the switch to OTC status is the concomitant drive by the pharmaceutical industry to increase lay awareness of the condition, particularly in countries such as the United States and New Zealand where direct-to-consumer advertising is legal. Self-screening tools are prevalent in this drive for disease recognition, and they frequently appeal to emotional rather than clinical imperatives.

Monistat (2023) provides an online symptom checker to promote its antifungal treatment. "Do you have a yeast infection?" asks the web page. "Do you have itching and irritation? Discharge?" The page underlines that "this symptom checker is not intended to be a diagnostic health tool. The actions and products it suggests do not constitute a medical diagnosis of a specific condition and do not take the place of the diagnosis or recommendations made by your physician." Yet it provides a "doctor discussion guide" for download and does make treatment recommendations.

Self-diagnosis is not driven by the pharmaceutical industry alone. Online communities—some funded by the industry, others not—also promote disease awareness. The Solve ME/CFS Initiative web page, for example, provides an interactive quiz to help an individual see whether they may have myalgic encephalomyelitis (ME) or chronic fatigue syndrome (CFS), albeit with the caution, "While we cannot provide medical advice, we hope this simple quiz, which is grounded in science, is useful" (2023). WebMD proposes a similar self-exploration with its page titled "Do I have Long Covid? Here's how to tell" (Levine 2022). While putatively medical advice, WebMD's business model is based on advertising revenues from pharma, hospitals, and other profit elements of the health care system.

The controversial nature of such diseases as CFS and long COVID helps to explain medical ambivalence, if not resentment, of lay prediagnosis (more on this in chapter 4). Until medicine officially sanctions particular conditions with a diagnostic label, it is reluctant to condone lay-driven disease campaigns (see P. Brown 1995).

By contrast, self-diagnosis appears to be welcome in certain well-defined circumstances. Already, the emphasis on self-care and "concordance" (rather than compliance) seeks to cast the layperson as a decision maker (Mullen 1997). Extending the autonomy of the individual beyond care to diagnosis, however, is more unusual. Outside of the discussion of vaginal yeast infection, self-diagnosis has its most robust supporters in those conditions for which medical assistance is not available, is unreliable, or is a burden to the public health system.

The extreme examples of malaria and altitude sickness are conditions that tend to surface in geographic locations where doctors are rarely found. Self-diagnosis becomes an imperative, or at least an aspiration. But the closer-to-home example of 2009–10 H1N1 influenza virus is perhaps pertinent. As mentioned above, self-diagnosis is a cornerstone of pandemic management. It falls under the category of "elimination of potential exposures," which is on the top level in the hierarchy of actions designed to minimize transmission of influenza (CDC 2009a). By minimizing outpatient visits for those with mild influenza-like illness, the self-diagnosed becomes self-isolated, concurrently reducing their opportunities to transmit the virus.

While this makes self-diagnosis of influenza highly desirable, no studies have confirmed its efficacy. The demedicalization of mild influenza presumes that individuals can distinguish among colds, influenza, pneumonia (or other lower respiratory infections), and other systemic illnesses. This may be correct, but it is untested. Researchers recently reported delays in treatment for potentially life-threatening illnesses that resulted from the incorrect diagnosis of influenza (Houlihan et al. 2010). Further, along with self-diagnosis comes self-treatment, and in many cases the rush toward oseltamivir (Tamiflu), which has been released in many countries as an OTC medication, creates the same commercial forces and potential conflicts as described above.

What makes this case interesting is that medicine has deemed self-diagnosis acceptable in this instance yet vigorously refutes its utility in lay-led, contested conditions where the consequences of misdiagnosis are arguably no more severe. This selective acceptance of self-diagnosis confirms the authoritative role of medicine, even while it enables individuals to decide for themselves what ails them. With respect to influenza infection, medicine remains the custodian of the diagnosis but determines who its delegates should be. Further, self-diagnosis presents challenges to the compliant "patient." While contemporary "consumers" may participate in their health care in new and autonomous ways, authorized self-diagnosis is nonetheless transformative and complex. As Henwood and colleagues' (2003) research shows, many individuals do not wish to assume responsibility for medical information and decision making. They indicate that it is the doctor's "job" and that ignorance about such matters is a relief rather than a source of disempowerment. Further, the skills required to seek, source, and appraise information are not within the ability, or even the interest, of all people. Finally, the nature of the doctor-patient relationship may not enable the enactment of an informed patient identity, particularly when the two are at odds.

There are no clear binaries to guide the incorporation of self-diagnosis into contemporary health management. It is a complex matter because it is a relational one, tightly bound up in the ways laypeople and doctors position themselves and interact with one another.

What Next?

"What is the place of the patient in the co-production of a diagnosis?" asks Blaxter (2009). In the presence of new technologies, must the patient vanish? Similarly, we should perhaps ask, "Where does the doctor go in this new era of the patient consumer-expert-advocate?"

New models for the doctor-patient relationship abound. They focus on partnerships (Williamson 1999); concordance (Mullen 1997); coprovision (Buetow 2005); interpretation (Leder 1990); negotiation; productive alliance (Filc 2006); homogilization (Buetow, Jutel, and Hoare 2009); or according to Shutzberg's metaphorical analysis, parent, partner, provider—or comrade (2020). The patient may be involved, expert, compliant, autonomous, or resourceful. But the majority of these models focus on transformation of the patient identity *within* the dominant biomedical model. Medicine is still the final authority, enabling patient participation, albeit on a short lead. "Expert patients" manage their own care: monitoring symptoms, using the appropriate treatment, optimizing their well-being, and generally managing their illness independently from the doctor (Wilson 2001). This patient expertise implies compliance with the medical model, including acceptance of medicine's definition of disease. Yet, as Julia Neuberger has noted, "active" and "patient" are contradictory terms (1999).

In spite of these changing dynamics, lay and expert knowledges retain their respective positions in the traditional hierarchy and give medicine the last word. This imbalance can explain the contested diagnoses that are discussed in the next chapter. It also explains why the integration of new players previously external to the doctor-patient relationship (such as technology and pharmaceutical firms, direct-to-consumer advertising, disease advocacy groups, and managed care) is experienced variably as introducing vulnerability and empowerment by doctors and patients alike. Nick Fox and Katie Ward's (2006) work on health identities is useful for understanding what is engendered by the changing status of patient and doctor in the diagnostic encounter: a paradox of both empowerment and disempowerment. Their empirical work reveals the blurring of identities in the independent patient, ranging from compliant to out-and-out rebellious, with the audacious "consumer" positioned somewhere in between. As health information flows across the internet, some consume it as an adjunct to medical care, seeking online communities in order to refine their knowledge, and become more expert in, say, the use of weight-loss medication. Discussing the ethnography of a weight-loss discussion list, Fox and Ward identify a group that sought to conform to biomedical expectations, incorporating medical opinion, specifically the opinion of users' individual general practitioners, to frame their activities. At the opposite extreme, women who have serious eating disorders used an online forum not to adhere to but rather to resist conventional medical treatment. The aim of that group was not to cure anorexia nervosa but to support individuals so diagnosed in circumventing the recommended medical approach.

Shutzberg (2021) proposes that the relationship between doctor and patient is mutually disempowering and turns to Patočka to muse on "a sentiment between former adversaries—a solidarity of the shaken" (236). She describes how doctor and patient unite against the absurdity of changes to eligibility for benefits, resisting together via the certification process to obtain the preferred outcome. They move from "adversaries to comrades in and through their common powerlessness" (241)

The technologies of diagnosis and the diagnoses themselves are neither prior nor independent. Fox and Ward's (2006) model, which is based on Gilles Deleuze and Felix Guattari's ontology, demonstrates the confluence of factors that creates the identity of the individual. It comprises an assemblage that cannot overlook the diagnosis. The identities of both doctor and patient are defined not only by each other but by the pivotal diagnosis that sits between both as explanation, expectation, trophy, stigmata, assault, confounder, justification, key, identifier, and so on.

Returning to Raymond Carver's poem, consider his interaction with his doctor. Imagine if the situation were a diagnosis other than catastrophic malignancy. There would still be a relational element in what the diagnosis means and how it is incorporated into the patient's experience of health and illness. "The X-ray is clear. There's nothing wrong." (*Are you sure? Am I imagining this? Is it in my head? Do you know what you are doing?*) "It's just a bit of airway irritation. Should clear up when the pollen levels drop." (*Damned trees! Maybe I'll go have a weekend on the coast. Thanks for the news. You been to the coast recently? Where'd you go?*) "You need to stretch yourself more. You're out of breath because you're getting unfit." (*Should be more disciplined. Should go to the gym. Used to go jogging—when did I get so lazy? How 'bout your waistline? Don't act so damned superior!*)

Diagnosis brings layperson and professional together in a curiously intimate and consequential way, with the goal of achieving a better understanding of a problematic state of being. The ideal encounter is explanatory, predictive, and curative. As illustrated in the pages to come, though, diagnosis can be both a disputed object and an integral component of health identity. In a contested diagnosis, there is both an individual and a collective disappointment, which chapter 4 explores.

CHAPTER FOUR

Contested Diagnoses and the Medically Unexplained

What happens when the chronically vulnerable person feels compelled to be a patient? The homeostasis of the chronic vulnerable state dissolves in a hunt for an elusive disease, a "monster that can be locked up with diagnosis." Months and even years pass, and no test result is sufficiently reproducible or specific to overwhelming uncertainty. The tragic patient is drowning in Bayesian false starts. Faced with escalating illness, so discordant from demonstrable disease, medicine is not likely to accept blame for subjecting the patient to months of an exercise that turned out to be flawed in design and iatrogenic in execution. One option is to suggest counseling of some ilk; more often than not, the patient hears, "You think it's in my mind," and bridles at the affront to their perspicacity, if not veracity. The battle is less likely to be joined if a diagnostic paralogism is offered; these are labels that subsume pathogenetic hypotheses. They promulgate a more vulnerable state by promising naught but palliation until an answer is forthcoming from science—sometime in the future.

NORTIN M. HADLER, MD (1996)

When Phil Brown first called for a sociology of diagnosis in his 1995 paper, "Naming and Framing," he used contested illness as the fulcrum of his argument. He claimed that it is precisely because lay and professional understandings of health and illness are different that the question of diagnosis is so important. The ways in which people experience illness do not necessarily align with the ways medical knowledge classifies disease: "Diagnostic discovery is frequently laden with dispute, which provides a lens for viewing many of the social conflicts which revolve around issues of medicine and health" (38).

I have written earlier about how medical authority may transform the patient narrative, rendering foreign what was once personal. This is most salient in the case of the contested diagnosis. A number of conditions—some common, others idiosyncratic—find their recognition thwarted by medicine. They are accepted neither by doctors nor by government or insurance companies, yet they are fully experienced by the individual as illness. This uncomfortable clash of perception is at the base of what is referred to as contested, or disputed, diseases. They are conditions that medicine does not acknowledge but sick persons—whether an individual or a group of individuals with what they consider the same condition—believe to be diseases. Sufferers often experience the defense of their illness as a battle, such as the one described by Nortin Hadler. His words punctuate the degree to which contest or dispute is always potentially present in the diagnostic process, particularly, as he notes here, in the case of the disability determination. The link to disability determination helps to explain dispute. It is linked with resource allocation, transforming the doctor into gatekeeper (rather than explainer), with diagnosis as a key.

In the pages that follow, we take a look at a few of the ways in which disease designation results in social conflict, likely to push the individual to contest a diagnosis or its absence. I then use the example of the medically unexplained symptom to demonstrate the discursive construction of illness that medicine cannot (or will not) currently label. Finally, I consider how the contest in lay-professional interactions may be receding, or at least changing. Here, my focus is mainly on collective discord. Where do lay and professional beliefs collide over what counts as a disease, and what responses do either party assume in the case of contest? But I also consider the importance that the diagnostic system confers to the epistemic setting of medicine, explaining in part, the tension that diagnosis, or its absence, presents to the sick person and to the doctor.

Dumit (2006) has defined five characteristics that link contested diagnoses. First, these diseases are frequently chronic. They do not fit the acute disease model and consequently, do not enable simple cost calculations. Second, they have uncertain etiology and are frequently "biomental," meaning their cause is attributed variably to physical, social, toxic-exposure, or psychiatric causes. Third, their treatment is diverse and may be approached by various therapeutic avenues, including alternative medicine. Fourth, their boundaries are unclear, and they have many comorbidities. While professionals might argue that they are psychogenic, patients might retort that their obvious depression is the result of the disregard in which they are held by the medical fraternity. Finally, they are "legally explosive," notably as a result of their link to disability assignment. If the conditions are not recognized as disease, sufferers are not entitled to compensation for treatment or for the changes the illnesses impose on their lifestyles.

Numerous conditions fit this bill. Fibromyalgia is one. It is a contested diagnosis of exclusion that may be proposed when a panoply of other potential medical explanations fail to explain chronic widespread pain, sleep disturbance, fatigue, and bilateral tender points. The etiology is uncertain, and it is indeed often referred to as psychogenic. There is no therapeutic agreement as to how fibromyalgia should be managed, and the diagnosis is clearly linked to disability allocation (Sim and Madden 2008).

In Sim and Madden's meta-synthesis of fibromyalgia studies, the pursuit of diagnosis emerges as one of the most pressing issues identified by sufferers of the condition. The symptoms they experienced were so incapacitating that they believed they must have undetected malignancy but were told by doctors that nothing was wrong and that their symptoms were psychological in nature, despite the distinctly physical manner in which they experienced them. They spoke of resentment for what they perceived to be a dismissive approach to their suffering. With fibromyalgia, receiving a diagnosis was initially a relief because it validated their illness, reassured them there was no malignancy, and gave them a sense of credibility lost in the prediagnosis process (Sim and Madden 2008).

In today's pandemic, COVID-19 is open to a similar contest. "Long COVID," or "long haul COVID," was initially viewed with some skepticism by the medical community. As Callard and Perego recount, the idea that COVID-19 symptoms would persist beyond the acute infectious period, and particularly in initially mild infections, was driven by advocacy from people suffering from ongoing symptoms weeks after their initial infection. To start with, the use of emphatic quotation marks, or the qualifier "so-called," in discussing long COVID in academic papers initially flagged the use of the term as somehow questionable. Today, "long COVID" has entered the lexicon (Callard and Perego 2021). But like fibromyalgia, Lyme disease, chronic fatigue, and many other enduring conditions, this extended experience of COVID-19 is in diagnostic flux. Those with the power to endorse it are eager to control even its discursive construction in advance of its diagnostic construction.

The status of long COVID is in constant transformation, given the recentness of its discovery. From its emergence in late 2019 until the submission of this manuscript in 2023, when I wrote about COVID-19, I needed to update myself frequently to keep up with the science but also with "discovery." Phil Brown (1995) maintains that discovery is not about biomedical facts; rather, it is "a set of understandings, relationships, and actions that are shaped by diverse kinds of knowledge, experience and power relations, and that are constantly in flux" (37). Long COVID thus serves as a kind of mega-example of the boundaries of diagnoses and the authority of medicine to acknowledge them. A diagnostic imperative drives both sick or disabled person and clinician toward diagnosis-as-closure. In the absence of a recognizable clinical diagnosis, the clinician will possibly attribute symptoms to mental disorder. Without a diagnosis, the illness is not legitimized, and the identity of the sick or disabled person is soiled. Rosenberg has written about the "tyranny of diagnosis," a tyranny to which these personal diagnosis projects are committed. What is needed is to put a name to troubles, or experiences of disablement. This can provide closure or a means by which to come to terms with dysfunction. What interpretation of troubles as pathologies may minimize in their translation as aspects of an individual's disease or disorder is the political or social framework in which such troubles are often fostered.

Not all diagnoses, however, are equal in the hierarchy of diagnoses, or what Dag Album refers to as "disease prestige." Diagnosees may believe they need to conceal particular diagnoses to avoid particular associations between diagnosis and character. The "lifestyle" diagnoses of diabetes, hypertension, and obesity, for example, are often associated with moral failing, that the diseases are the result of gluttony or sloth. The implication that one has a disorder one should be able to "do something" about makes certain labels more welcome than others.

Contest is accentuated by the latent dichotomy between illness and disease, the unequal power relationship between the patient and doctor, and the need for a medical diagnosis before other services can be accessed. Contest, notably in emerging illnesses such as fibromyalgia above, assumes a particularly acute form when the absence of diagnosis denies the patient access to the sick role and (more importantly) to institutional recognition of suffering. Many have written of the distress of patients who do not receive a diagnosis for their complaint. This distress typically focuses on disorder, confusion, and fear of service denial or of being stigmatized by a psychogenic explanation (de Boer and Slatman 2023; Dumit 2006; Malterud 2001, 2005; Nettleton 2006).

Dumit (2006) describes how conflict is shaped both within and outside of the patient-doctor relationship. Clinicians are directed in their practice by the impositions of the health maintenance organization, the employer, and the insurer; bureaucracy determines who can provide care and for which ailments. These organizations, combined, have symbolic domination over the individual patient. But the key point, as Dumit makes clear in this and other papers, is "the intense interplay between diagnosis and legitimacy: without a diagnosis and other forms of acceptance into the medical system, sufferers are at risk of being denied social recognition of their very suffering and accused of simply faking it" (578).

Contested diagnoses are typically those that cannot currently be explained by medicine or whose explanations are in dispute (Brown and Zavestoski 2004). The contest focuses on debate around whether they are primarily social, psychiatric, or biological (Dumit 2006). These are illnesses that "are not defined in terms of organic pathology, but on the basis of their symptoms" (Nettleton et al. 2004). I discuss, overleaf, how the medical literature deals with medically unexplained, enigmatic symptoms. For the patient, the difficulty of living with the uncertainty of non-diagnosis, and of defending the legitimacy of complaints, results in significant distress and dissatisfaction with the medical profession (Nettleton 2006).

Conversely, conflict may also arise when diagnosis achieves nonclinical ends and therefore stymies the rights of patients who do not believe themselves to be ill. A powerful example is political psychiatry, where dissent is treated as mental illness. Robin Munro quotes a Chinese textbook that develops the notion of "political mania" as a form of paranoid psychosis: "Those afflicted do avid research into politics and put forward a whole set of original theories of their own, which they then try to peddle by every means possible . . . such people are sometimes viewed [by others] as being political dissidents" (*Sifa jingshen yixue jianding zixun jieda*, in Munro 2002). During the Cultural Revolution in China, the Revolutionary Committee oversaw psychiatry and its diagnostic practices, requiring political justification of diagnostic and treatment decision making of mental health patients (Yip 2005).

Similar political control of diagnostic categories figures in Russian psychiatry. Coercive psychiatry was widely used well into the 1980s to hospitalize political and religious dissidents, in the absence of psychiatric illness. What enabled this detention were laws that allowed medical custody of individuals who had committed a crime but were "nonimputable" because of mental illness. Antipsychotic medication was used in high doses to treat "delusions of reformism" and "anti-Soviet thoughts" (Bonnie 2002, 137–38).

Lest readers be misled that the politicization of diagnosis is restricted to repressive regimes, the more conventional diagnoses of antisocial personality disorder (APD) and dangerous and severe personality disorder (DSPD) bear mentioning. As Corbett and Westwood (2005) point out, many of the diagnostic criteria for APD as cited in the *DSM-IV* are typical within particular subcultures and actually emerge as a result of alienation from dominant norms and values (e.g., failure to conform to social norms, deceitfulness/lying, failure to plan ahead, irritability or aggressiveness, disregard for safety, failure to sustain consistent work or pay debts, and lack of remorse regarding hurting or stealing from another, among individuals at least 18 years of age) (124–25).

DSPD is a diagnosis that, argue Corbett and Westwood (2005), emerges from a risk-averse society, anxious to provide a perception of safety in the context of a highly sensationalized debate about the relationship between psychiatric diseases and violence. In this case, the idea that individuals may present a risk to social order above and beyond the preexisting health laws is embodied in the diagnosis.

Medically Unexplained Symptoms

The issue of the non-diagnosable medical complaint takes a curious role, challenging medicine's modus operandi, which seeks to identify and treat disease. Where medicine is not able to label a patient's affliction within its available diagnostic frameworks, its discursive approach reveals much about how medicine considers conditions that are baffling or not easily classified.

The phrase "medically unexplained symptoms" would seem self-explanatory. There are physical symptoms that bring patients to consult but for which doctors cannot establish a cause. The discursive approach of both medical literature and practice is paradoxical—transforming the range of unexplained causes for consultation into a unitary condition with its own diagnostic label, linking it to psychiatric dysfunction, augmenting patient suffering, and failing to appraise critically the limitations of its episteme. In the following pages, I make that critical appraisal, reviewing the role of the symptom, assessing the current literature that focuses on the medically unexplained symptom, and identifying how medical discourses about medically unexplained symptoms shift responsibility for illness to the patient and interfere with the interpretative role of the doctor.

The Symptom

Foucault (1963) describes how the symptom took on a new role in nineteenth-century clinical medicine. Previously the sole locus of medical interest, it became instead a key, a clue, or a pointer to deeper and more significant conditions. This is what the taxonomists and the nosologists were attempting to clarify as they assembled symptoms into diagnostic classifications. The arrangement of symptoms was a window to otherwise hidden disease. "Cough, chest pain and shortness of breath are not pleurisy . . . they are its essential symptoms," writes Foucault (89, translation mine). No longer were symptoms considered as individual phenomena; they became the external expression of disease. This transformed the role of doctor into one of detective: unscrambling the messages of the symptom to discover the link between signifier and pathology.

Drew Leder (1990) describes this stealth work as an interpretive process. The patient brings to the medical consultation a situation that they are not fully able to interpret but have assigned to the medical realm. In their desire to understand the discomfort, the cough, the rash, the swelling, or the cramp, they initiate an encounter with the doctor. This is what the doctor will refer to as the symptom: a "subjective" experience or change in function. In turn, the doctor channels the narrative of illness or dysfunction toward an interpretive outcome, asking questions about personal and family history, querying both the presentation and absence of symptoms. The doctor then undertakes a physical assessment, exploring the body-object—now silent while palpated, auscultated, and measured—to create a narrative that explains the patient's complaint. And finally, both patient and doctor acquiesce to the numerical findings contained in instrumental texts such as X-ray, scans, blood count, or manometer.

This encounter is guided by a presumptive paradigm and measured by clinical efficacy. This means that prediagnosis conceptions underpin the manner by which the doctor explores the complaint and prevent an aimless "fishing trip" of non-systematic explorations and questions. The collection of symptoms, along with the patient's story, points the doctor in a particular direction, suggesting a bouquet of potential diagnoses or explanations and reducing the complexity of decision making (Croskerry 2002). It also means that the encounter cannot be considered successful if medical interpretation emerging from the interaction does not result in the patient's cooperative comprehension or in clinical improvement.

Yet, anywhere from 10 to 35 percent of primary consultations fail to alleviate the presenting complaint. Frustrated by symptoms for which they cannot find a recognized medical diagnosis, doctors devote much energy to explaining and identifying a presumed root cause. This entails a significant financial and structural impact on health care, generates inappropriate referrals and treatment, engenders physician frustration, and of course, results in distress for the patient, who generally consults with the hope of identifying an explanation and concordant cure.

The term "medically unexplained symptom" and its impact is the subject of increasing reflection in the medical literature. A critical review of articles focusing on these enigmatic symptoms demonstrates a growing concern with the burden that they present for patients, doctors and the health care system, but it also reveals a curious approach to the problem (Jutel 2010). Paradoxically, many of the articles resort to creating a catchall diagnostic category in which to place the unexplained.* The phrase "medically unexplained symptoms" is frequently used interchangeably with psychiatric diagnostic terms, such as somatoform disorder, somatizing, or functional somatic syndrome, that imply psychogenic or sociogenic origin. The medically unexplained symptom is an important diagnostic component of these conditions, but in these articles they are subsumed within the psychiatric disorders and used synonymously. A modest proportion of these articles, however, critique the tendency to provide a psychogenic explanation, to diagnose by exclusion, or to obscure the limitations of medical knowledge vis-à-vis the physical complaints of patients. I discuss this in greater length below.

But whether the publications see medically unexplained symptoms as psychogenic or not, there is a pervasive reference to them as an entity or as a unified condition that could be considered under one light. The literature links medically unexplained symptoms semantically with phrases such as "the *problem* of medically unexplained symptoms," "*diagnosing* medically unexplained symptoms," "*treating* medically unexplained symptoms." This semantic formulation reduces chronic fatigue, lower back pain, irritable bowel syndrome, and so on to the unitary label of medically unexplained symptoms. The use of the acronym MUS reifies the notion that all physical complaints without explanation can be viewed in the same way. But it is not just nomenclature. References to medically unexplained symptoms as a *diagnosis*, a *problem* to be approached epidemiologically, a treatable or preventable *condition*, and to suf-

---

* This approach may be paradoxical, but it is not surprising. Medicine has had a variety of historical mechanisms for arranging that which does not fit into current nosology, from reflex theory to spinal irritation, hysteria, dissociation, and others (Shorter 1992).

ferers as a homogenous group, confirm that this is an approach that reasons through diagnosis rather than interpretation.

Psychiatry to Explain the Unexplainable

Rosenberg (2006) writes that "psychiatry is the residuary legatee of . . . developments that have always been contested at the ever-shifting boundary between disease and deviance, feeling and symptom, the random and the determined, the stigmatized and the value-free" (237). He seeks here to account for how disease categories explain behavior and emotional pain. This is relevant to the issue of medically unexplained symptoms, as the seemingly unjustified symptoms are "behaviors" in a model that uses psychiatry to explain the unexplained. This psychiatric domiciliation of the unexplained is problematic because it frequently relies on diagnosis by exclusion (settled upon by ruling out other explanations), fails to acknowledge the limitations of knowledge, and shifts responsibility for cause and cure in a way that ignores sociohistorical realities (as we see below).

First, considering medically unexplained symptoms a psychiatric disorder is a diagnosis by exclusion. In other words, it is a diagnosis that is made not on the basis of what it is but on the basis of what it is not. The absence of explanation, rather than the presence of a well-defined feature, is pathognomic of the condition. The label becomes a wastebasket diagnosis, a classification in which may be placed many conditions that don't easily fit elsewhere. As Robins and Helzer (1986) point out, psychiatric diagnosis is already challenged by the absence of definitive tests to mark the presence of a disorder; there is no equivalent to the X-ray of orthopedics or the hemoculture of infectious disease. It is therefore difficult to establish a positive diagnosis yet facile to attach a positive psychiatric diagnosis to a medical patient.

Second, this assumption of psychiatric disorder in the absence of other diagnoses presumes the infallibility of the doctor and of the field. And yet one postmortem study revealed discrepancies in major diagnoses of 39 percent and of minor diagnoses in 50 percent of cases (Aalton et al. 2006). There are numerous diagnostic errors that can be retrospectively assigned to an incomplete knowledge of the field. For example, Lyme disease, prior to its designation as a specific diagnosable entity, was often cast as atypical rheumatoid arthritis (Graber et al. 2002). Multiple sclerosis was frequently diagnosed as a psychiatric disorder, possibly because many early symptoms are subjective (Walzl,

Solomon, and Stone 2022) and may also be atypical, presenting challenges for clinician and patient alike (Malterud and Taksdal 2007).

Advances in genetic understandings of illness provide links between pathologies that were previously seen as completely distinct (Miller 2006). As Kirmayer and colleagues (2004) state, "The lack of explanation reflects the limits of medical knowledge, available technology and the epistemological difficulties of assigning a clear cause to subjective complains like pain and fatigue, which may have no objectively measurable correlates and may change rapidly over time in quality and intensity."

Third, positing the cause for the unexplained symptom as the patient's mental health shifts responsibility for the failure to explain the symptom from the doctor to the patient. Hadler (1996) reflects upon both causes and limitations of this catchall psychogenic labeling, describing medicine as "not [being] likely to accept blame for subjecting the patient to months of an exercise that turn[s] out to be flawed in design and iatrogenic in execution." Similarly, Nettleton (2006) reports that the effort of trying to palliate symptoms in the absence of a diagnosis is as onerous as the symptoms themselves. "Society does not readily give people permission to be ill," she writes, "in the absence of an 'accepted' abnormal pathology or physiology."

Pilowsky (1994) claims that the contest of diagnosis is weighted toward the physician. He defines abnormal illness behavior as an "inappropriate or maladaptive mode of experiencing . . . one's own state of health which persists despite the fact that an appropriate social agent . . . has an accurate and reasonably lucid explanation of the nature of the person's health status" (568). He does point out that the doctor's potential to err is an important liability of this definition and that in some cases there is a hasty progression from lack of explanation to considering a patient's behavior "abnormal." Salient in Pilowsky's definition is the recognition of the important, yet equivocal, role of the "social agent," or doctor.

Locating the symptom in psychology ascribes responsibility and moral blame in a way that encourages patient resistance (Kirmayer et al. 2004). While a physical explanation for a symptom confers, in most cases, a lack of personal responsibility for its onset, a psychiatric one implies that the patient might have the ability to both control and reverse the physical symptoms, an interpretation that may seem impossible to the sufferer and brings with it stigma and shame.

And finally, this psychogenic explanation relies for diagnostic criteria upon historically and socially developed patterns of behavior that emerge from the expectations of modern medicine. An important criterion in the "diagnosis" of MUS (acronym use intentional) is frequency of general practitioner (GP) attendance. Against the background I have introduced above, repeated consultations for complaints that have no readily visible disease explanation may be the result of compliance with social expectations about the role of the doctor and of medicine.

For example, parents are rewarded for medicalizing their children's health: many countries provide financial or other incentives for "well-child" checkups. Direct-to-consumer advertising admonishes the public to "check with your doctor and find out if X is right for you!" using enticing and effective models to elicit consumption of medical care generally and of pharmaceutical products specifically. General medical practice may include such nonmedical services as family planning and ear piercing. Women are far greater consumers of these services than men and are more often subject to, and compliant with, calls to consult the doctor, resulting in a greater prevalence of "diagnosed" MUS. This compliance is historically learned from the medicalization of women's health, as contained in (but not restricted to) menstrual disability theory. Based on the Newtonian concept that energy can neither be created nor destroyed, this approach to women's health, originating in the nineteenth century, held that women's periodic bleeding represented the loss of vital energy (Vertinsky 1994). Because women were "eternally injured," they were transformed into docile subjects who sought medical attention readily. Subsequently, they become unequally slotted into the category of psychiatric illness by exclusion. Malterud's work submits that clinical approach is based on gender and detrimentally traps women in diagnostic categories and treatment protocols (Malterud 1999, 2000, 2001; Malterud, Candid, and Code 2004).

Health promotion organizations, in contrast, lament the noncompliance of men, who are less likely than women to see their doctor regularly. A growing body of literature points out that men have poor help-seeking behavior, are reluctant to consult a GP until well past the propitious time (Galdas, Cheater, and Marshall 2005), and are more reliant on social factors than on the gravity of symptoms to determine when they will consult (Wolters et al. 2002). Poor help-seeking behavior is proposed as one of the reasons for worse health outcomes in men than in women (Galdas, Cheater, and Marshall 2005). Addressing this deficiency is an important focus of men's health initiatives (McKinlay 2005). Since men are often reluctant to consult their GP, alternatives have been developed, including using sports clubs and pubs as venues for health promotion activities.

How Then to Explain the Unexplained?

I have shown the limitations of "diagnosing" medically unexplained symptoms as an entity. It is a diagnosis of exclusion that presumes the infallibility of the physician and the omniscience of medicine. It transfers responsibility for the disorder to the patient, and it ignores sociohistorical practices that influence patient behavior and place women unequally under scrutiny for psychogenic disorder.

There is, however, a range of explanations for complaints that are not linked with disease. Returning to Leder's hermeneutic contextualization of the patient-doctor encounter, we can easily see that one is that the patient has incorrectly attributed the origin of their complaint to the realm of medicine. Leder describes what he calls the "experiential text" that consists of the experiences that the person has identified as significant and disruptive. While this experiential text may not legitimately have its explanation in medicine, medicine's role as arbitrator may lead the patient to presume the contrary. And, as industry marketing uses the stamp of medical approval to sell its wares, it is increasingly likely that the patient will assume their problems are medical (Conrad and Leiter 2004).

Many serious symptoms and dysfunctions affecting digestion, mobility, comfort, and kinesthesia may be quite clearly "real" without being medical. The tortuous course of lower back pain in the absence of structural pathology may be explained by a muscle-balance assessment and "cured" by development of core strength and exercise prescription, rather than surgical or medical or pharmacological solutions (Abenhaim et al. 2000). Similarly, bloating, flatulence, diarrhea, and other digestive system distress that cannot be explained by celiac disease or other defined clinical entity may still be related to dietary intolerances and obscure food allergies that a nutritionist could better address or that the person themselves could resolve by trial and error (see, for example, Meador's [2005] unusual case study of a specific brand of toothpaste as a causative factor in intractable diarrhea). A biomechanical explanation may be at the heart of many functional disorders that an occupational therapist, clinical biomechanist, or podiatrist would be better suited than either a physician or surgeon to diagnose and correct.

In the same way, unknown and unexpected environmental factors may explain any number of respiratory, gastroenteric, cutaneous, and functional symptoms. Many conditions that are medically unexplained overlap strongly with explained conditions, such as asthma. Environmental factors are an underresearched area of potential causation and are often contested diagnoses, reflecting sociopolitical forms of illness in the case of unacknowledged environmental contamination, for example (Brown 1995; Kipen and Fiedler 2002).

A condition may be medical but not recognized as such. Inclusion in the *ICD* is by application. A condition must be first recognized, and then championed, to be considered. Some conditions are functional and treatable but are not linked to a particular pathology. Radiotherapy damage, whiplash sequelae, and even the common cough (A. Goldstein 2007) can be discrete entities of their own that we could perhaps understand as physical dysfunctions rather than as diseases.

And finally, we need to consider that the explanation *may* be psychiatric. Physical symptoms are recognized as part of psychiatric syndromes. They are a common comorbidity in major depressive disorder (Arnow et al. 2006), are part of the diagnostic criteria for generalized anxiety, are often linked with psychosis, and so on. Psychiatry is a legitimate form of medicine and has a diagnostic framework for disease, as does physical medicine. This should not, however, be a diagnosis by exclusion; it should be based on positive findings in the context of a comprehensive biopsychosocial assessment.

Disease Discovery

I have stressed that classification is a human endeavor that involves parceling a continuum of nature into discrete packages that make sense to those who are in the business of differentiating the particular conditions at hand. How then does a disease come to be classified? The way a particular set of symptoms becomes accepted as one thing and not another must be part of how we understand diagnosis and its impact. This is what Brown (1995) refers to as the "disease discovery process."

Brown proposes a model for disease discovery. Unlike other models (for example, Conrad and Schneider's [1980] model of medicalization), Brown's provides a mechanism for understanding the roles that laypeople and the medical institution, respectively, play in the establishment of diagnoses, including those where lay and professional views might not agree. His model identifies distinct factors that are typically part of the disease discovery process, though not present in all disease discovery, and are not sequential. They do, in any case, demonstrate how consensus, politics, and interest must converge before a diagnostic category can exist. There are four elements in Brown's model: lay discovery, social movement, professional factors, and institutional and organizational factors.

Whether a disease is contested will depend on the degree to which, as discussed above, laypeople and medicine agree upon the nature of a particular condition. This agreement in turn, is likely to be influenced by a range of factors, as described by Dumit in the earlier pages of this chapter. How unusual is the symptomatology? What are the treatment regimens? Can the condition be cast as psychogenic? Are there resources at stake?

The histories of individual diseases illustrate how these factors interact to generate diagnoses.* Wilbur Scott provides a detailed account of post-traumatic stress disorder's (PTSD) incorporation into the *DSM-III*: considerable individual and collective labor was required to obtain acknowledgment that the psychological distress of numerous Vietnam veterans was distinct from the psychosis, cowardice, or malingering, to which it had previously been attributed (1990). The effort was political, involving negotiation, relationship management, and persuasion. Scott recounts this as an example of how diagnosis brings conditions forward as "always-already-there objects in the world" via a convincing display of objective evidence: "a discovery of what was present but previously unseen" (295). The agents in this particular political process were cognizant that it did not suffice for the condition to be, as they saw it, a real thing in the world; those with control over classificatory processes needed to be made to face the realness of the diagnosis. This could only be accomplished by concerted and repeated efforts. Choosing how to speak of the disorder, with whom to discuss it, when to have discussions, and how to use collective action were instrumental factors in the campaign to incorporate PTSD into the *DSM-III*.

Wilbur Scott's (1990) description brings to the fore each step in Brown's (1995) model of social discovery. Lay discoveries by individual veterans, buttressed by the social movement of veteran organizations, were pivotal in the

---

* A number of publications explore the histories of particular diseases, many of which are useful for punctuating the contexts in which these diseases emerged and gained purchase, including, among others, Aronowitz 1998; Horwitz and Wakefield 2007; Packard et al. 2004; Rosenberg and Golden 1992.

acceptance of PTSD in the *DSM-III*. Prior to its introduction as a diagnosis, there was an acknowledged interest in the psychiatric casualties of combat, both immediate and delayed. In the Vietnam era, though, despite the frequent clinical observation and reports of deeply stressed veterans, there was no classification in the *DSM* that met the description of their distress or that included the war experience as part of the diagnostic pathway.

The development of a post-combat stress disorder was to emerge from a combination of lay and professional forces committed to the welfare of returning military personnel. As Brown notes is to be expected in lay-led discovery, the promotion of this particular label required professional backing. Robert Lifton and Chaim Shatan, both psychiatrists with strong antiwar sentiment, joined the Vietnam Veterans Against the War (VVAW) "rap sessions." These meetings had a political purpose of consolidating and disseminating information about the horrors of the war to the public but also provided an opportunity for a kind of street-corner psychiatry that enabled Lifton and Shatan to witness and gather information about a post-Vietnam syndrome (W. Scott 1990).

At almost the same time the *DSM-III* revisions were being undertaken, news of the demedicalization of homosexuality opened the way for the introduction of many other changes to the diagnostic manual. Shatan, Lifton, and Sarah Haley, a Veterans Administration (VA) social worker whose own family history of exposure to war atrocities made her particularly sensitive to the reports of her patients, joined with the director of the National Veterans Resource Project to launch a working group on post-combat disorder. This lay-professional working group devoted itself to gathering empirical evidence of the disorder and to enlisting the political support of personalities in the psychiatric community (notably Robert Spitzer). Their work was successful, and in 1978, the Committee on Reactive Disorders of the American Psychiatric Association recommended the diagnostic label of "post-traumatic stress disorder" (Scott 1990).

Gulf War–related illnesses—like chronic fatigue syndrome, multiple chemical sensitivity, and fibromyalgia—serve as an example of medically unexplained symptoms as well as an example of lay activism playing an important role in disease recognition. As many as 70,000 Gulf War veterans have sought treatment for illnesses that they believe are the result of exposure to environmental hazards during service (Zavestoski et al. 2002). They have reported such symptoms as nausea, loss of concentration, irritable bowels, and blurred vision. Two conflicting explanations are presented to explain these symptoms: on the one hand, exposure to environmental hazards, such as anti-nerve-gas pills, nerve agents such as sarin, pesticides, insect repellents, and smoke from oil fires, tent heaters, and the burning of human waste; but on the other, traumatic psychological stress (Proctor et al. 1998).

The Department of Veterans Affairs initially denied care for such ailments on the basis that the symptoms were not diagnosable, maintaining that they were the result of stress, not of toxic exposure (Zavestoski et al. 2002). A National Institutes of Health technology workshop concluded that veteran illnesses were caused by PTSD that manifested through "somatic and multisystem symptoms" (NIH 1994, in Zavestoski et al. 2002). Veterans resisted this label, partly because it did not necessarily guarantee access to services and treatment. Veterans also found it a convenient distraction for the Department of Defense from the potential environmental exposures and, by extension, from their own liability. They continued to push for more research into potential environmental hazards (Zavestoski et al. 2002). Gulf War veterans framed their inability to get the recognition and treatment they were entitled to as an injustice, drawing on the experiences of Vietnam vets who were exposed to Agent Orange (Brown and Zavestoski 2004).

Veterans began to speak out, and increased media coverage resulted in collective mobilization. In 1994, the VA began providing care as a consequence of legislation requiring benefits for all chronically disabled veterans with undiagnosed disease. Despite this, many veterans still thought they were not getting the care they deserved (Zavestoski et al. 2002). Many felt betrayed by the government's refusal to provide them treatment and its insistence that there was not enough science to support their claims.

The veterans' actions are an example of health social movements (HSM), an important political force that challenges political power, professional authority, and personal and collective identity. Specifically, these movements address access to or provision of health services; the experiences of disease, illness, and disability, particularly contested illness; and health inequality and inequalities related to ethnicity, race, gender, class, sexuality. The way HSMs operate has been influenced by an era of scientization. HSMs engage with medical science and public health to encourage favorable research, utilize resources, and produce their own knowledge. The movements are thus attempting to democratize the production of knowledge in order to challenge traditional

assumptions about causation and prevention, thus engaging more successfully in policy advocacy (Brown and Zavestoski 2004).

One figuration of the health social movement is the embodied health movement (EHM), which is organized to achieve medical recognition for a particular illness/disease, along with treatment and research. Embodied health movements challenge science on etiology, diagnosis, treatment, and prevention by
mobilizing medical professionals and scientists. Other examples of embodied
health movements include the breast cancer, AIDS, and tobacco control movements (Brown and Zavestoski 2004). The experience of those with the disease
plays an important role. AIDS activists, for example, became experts on the
illness and were then able to have a significant influence on the production
of knowledge, thus shaping policies and influencing research into treatments
(Epstein 1996).

The exemplar EHM is the environmental breast cancer movement. Breast
cancer was constructed as a problem of insufficient knowledge, not a stigma
or a problem of access to quality treatment. This linked breast cancer to institutional and governmental neglect and a failure to prioritize research funds.
Activists successfully articulated their issues to the general public and politicians through media coverage of the movement's activities. Breast cancer was
subsequently constructed not as an individual problem but as a crisis for the
general public. This was done by using three sets of culturally resonant frames,
in both the media and congressional hearings. First, breast cancer was framed
as an epidemic; second, it was framed as a problem of gender equity; and third,
it was framed as a threat to families (Kolker 2004).

In contrast, the discovery of Alzheimer disease was not lay initiated but
owes its current position in public awareness to lay efforts. Alzheimer disease,
which was named in the early twentieth century, was promoted by neurological researchers, and lay participation played a much later role, notable for the
promotion of the diagnosis rather than for its creation. Scientific advancement,
interprofessional relationships, and a particular cultural context enabled the
discovery of this now renowned diagnosis.

Two different neuropathological schools (in Munich, where Alzheimer worked
in Kraepelin's laboratory, and in Prague where Fischer worked under Pick) were
involved in a range of discoveries that were to frame Alzheimer disease. Previous medical literature described dementia in purely clinical terms and linked
it with normal aging. The introduction of new staining and autopsy results en-

abled Alzheimer and his colleagues to identify "neurofibrillary tangles." Simultaneously, presumably using similar technology, Fischer described "senile plaques." Both lesions are characteristic of what we call Alzheimer disease today. But scientific rivalry between the schools at Munich and at Prague, and between Alzheimer and Fischer, resulted in a range of explanatory claims and descriptions for these disorders, including Fischer's plaques, Fischer's presbyophenia, and of course, the now-assimilated Alzheimer disease (Amaducci et al. 1986).

The nosological discussion was resolved not by technological advances but by Kraepelin, the director of the department in which Alzheimer worked. Kraepelin was a researcher whose own work was devoted to the classification of psychiatric disorders and disease categories. He assigned his junior's name to the diagnosis of presenile dementia. Amaducci et al. (1986) surmises that this action was taken to consolidate the position both of Kraepelin's school and of his researcher, and comments that Kraepelin's reputation and authority were of primary importance in the creation and perpetuation of this particular diagnosis. It is safe to presume that Kraepelin's particular focus on taxonomy (see Kahn 1957) may have contributed to his interest and success in assigning the name to the condition.

Patrick Fox (1989) further maintains that the context of medicine at the time of these discoveries enabled the creation of this diagnosis. Alzheimer believed that the changes he saw in the brain tissue were due to more than just aging: "The elimination of the age criterion was central because it contributed to the transformation of what had been generally considered 'senility' into a specific disease with specific pathological characteristics and symptoms" (59). Fox also describes the push from family members of Alzheimer patients, which, from the mid-twentieth century, rallied behind the Alzheimer disease label to bring it forward in public consciousness, generate research interest, and promote its diagnostic status as well as its characterization as a leading cause of death.

Many other diseases, however, remain in flux, perceived as medical diseases to lay sufferers but not accepted as such by medicine. They are in the throes of being variably discovered or discarded. As Brown (1995) has also pointed out, the degree to which medicine might resist the incorporation of a condition as diagnosis depends on innumerable factors. Iatrogenicity, stigma, stereotypes, and corporate responsibility are all barriers to lay-led disease-recognition campaigns.

Whose Diagnosis?

Numerous pressures are chipping away at medicine's authority to diagnose. Whether this reduces or increases contest is to be seen. I discuss them in greater depth in other chapters, but I draw some of them back in here for the purpose of exploring how these pressures contribute to a changing balance in the diagnostic contest.

First, there is a distinct change in the lay-professional relationship discussed in chapter 3. Buetow, Jutel, and Hoare (2009) have labeled the evolving roles lay and medical practitioner play in their interactions as homologization, or a role convergence with reduced social distances between doctors and patient. Wider access to medical information has fueled changes in this relationship, where mutually accessed information may converge. At the same time, differences persist, and the wider access to information also allows for wider access to pharmaceutical marketing influence (not always ethical) and to alternatives forms of expertise, some considered questionable by the medical establishment.

This is not to say that medicine no longer has authority. The biomedical expertise of those trained to practice medicine still carries much weight. The practice of medicine, as well as its authority, is socially contingent, framed by broader sociotechnological change (Nettleton 2004). Nettleton discusses this change, in particular about the informatization of medicine, where the body is seen as a system of information networks: the art of medicine gives way to evidence-based practice, the physical body defers to the CT scan, information once restricted to medicine is now available to the lay web-surfer, and the doctor-patient relationship becomes a meeting of experts.

Second, medicine's jurisdiction is shifting, incorporating new agents and social forces in its contemporary context. Among them, as we shall see in greater depth in chapter 6, are commercial agents, such as the pharmaceutical industry. Linked to this industry, and in the context of increased lay engagement with medical information, is the trend toward self-diagnosis.

Many pharmaceutical marketing websites provide a range of tools to encourage the individual to diagnose themselves and to present the diagnosis to the doctor and request the recommended treatment. The tools may include simple descriptions in lay language of features of a particular disease, checklists of risk factors, symptom diaries, and other online symptom assessment tests. This approach fits in neatly with the previously described increasing role of the patient in the doctor-patient encounter. Encouraging the patient to pre-identify specific conditions prior to consulting the doctor is an important cornerstone of the disease branding strategies that seek to drive the market to recognize the presence of disease more widely and direct both patients and caregivers in the way they see particular pathologies.

As we have seen in chapter 3, self-diagnosis is not yet held in high regard by the medical profession and is considered useful only in certain circumstances. There seem to be two situations in which self-diagnosis is condoned by medicine. The first is where there is a public health imperative, that is to say, where population health is likely to be improved if laypeople are able to diagnose either a contagious or a serious disease (and where early detection contributes to reduced morbidity). This was certainly the case with COVID-19 and the use of rapid antigen testing and self-isolation (see Petersen and Pienarr 2024). The second is with common benign disorders. Where practitioners consistently draw the line in their tolerance of self-diagnosis is when it presents as what Barsky and Borus (1999) refer to as "embattled advocacy," or self-diagnosis as a gesture of defiance to critique the judgment of the doctor. These authors describe a "self-perpetuating, self-validating cycle in which common, endemic, somatic symptoms are incorrectly attributed to serious abnormality, reinforcing the patient's belief that he or she has a serious disease" (910), usually around conditions like fibromyalgia or chronic fatigue that the medical establishment is yet to explain satisfactorily and for which candidate explanations abound in online health communities.

Diagnosis offers a tool for political engagement in response to the rejection of disease claims. Diagnoses such as PTSD, black lung, and environmental disease offer social recognition for victims of abuse or toxic exposure, opening the door to care and to compensation (Brown 1995). Diagnosis also provides a focus for a growing number of internet communities. Web pages play a part in the social health movement, gathering individuals around existing and emerging diseases, both contested and accepted. These internet communities offer an alternative support structure when the absence of diagnosis impugns the medical legitimacy of the individual's complaint (Dumit 2006). These communities "create their own separate and distinct medical culture, a culture that gives primary importance to the role of subjective experience" (D. Goldstein 2004, 127). Examples of virtual communities creating an alternative culture are the pro-anorexia sites that seek to redefine anorexia nervosa outside of medical discourse, casting it instead as a sanctuary, a "place where control and purity [can] be found" (Fox, Ward, and O'Rourke 2005, 958). Conversely,

internet communities are also launched by health providers who have identified web pages as a site at which patients can be transformed from consumers
into a "community of practice" with potentially improved health outcomes
(Winkelman and Choo 2003).

In a general sense, virtual communities provide a sanctuary for alternative
and stigmatized groups. Notable for their genesis in medical-lay discord about
diagnosis, these groups may, on the one hand, provide support for illnesses
that medicine does not sanction. On the other hand, they may reject diagnostic classification, seeking to redefine what medicine perceives as disease in
other terms (for example, see St-Onge's team on psychosis [2005]). Or they may
accept diagnosis but reject the curtailing of what are more generally seen as
undesirable symptoms. The Hearing Voice Network seeks a nonmedical solution to the voices heard (and usually chemically repressed) by people who are
diagnosed with psychotic diseases (Sheffield Hearing Voices Network 2010).

Diagnostic Uncertainty

In parallel with the medically unexplained, we also find the vexed diagnostically "uncertain." Just as with "unexplained," this seemingly banal term takes
on an interesting other twist that adds to the tension about diagnosis, its importance, who gets to make it, and how it will organize the experience of
dysfunction.

The term "diagnostic uncertainty" is being used increasingly in medical
practice to indicate conditions for which a doctor, or doctors in general, are
unable to provide a diagnosis. This is to say, the term is deployed not (as the
words themselves would suggest) to indicate a situation of confusion, where
there are a number of possible outcomes; rather, it designates something for
which there is no obvious diagnosis. There is a conflation of the unknown and
the uncertain that, I have argued in depth elsewhere (see Jutel 2021), is one of
the ways that medicine protects its diagnostic system.

If diagnosis is the underpinning framework for medicine, then to be a medical problem is to be diagnosable. What happens when something isn't? To be
clear, in the early days of scientific medicine, it was diagnosis that set medicine apart from myriad other healing approaches. It remains a carefully guarded
means by which medicine protects its position at the summit of the health
professional hierarchy. Few other professions are entitled to diagnose, and when
they are, the privilege is carefully guarded. A nurse practitioner or a physiotherapist can diagnose in carefully circumscribed areas of dysfunction, but

only because medicine said it was OK. It is the diagnosis that protects the jurisdictional boundaries of medicine.

Yet the system fails from time to time. Medical knowledge has its limitations. Owen Whooley has argued that it is only by shedding light on how groups deal the failures of their systems, and the limitations of their specific fields of knowledge and knowledge tools, that we can truly understand their paradigms, practices, and politics.

I see the use of the terms "diagnostic uncertainty" and "medically unexplained symptoms" as a powerful way that medicine justifies its shortcomings. It is a sort of *epistemic defense*, that is to say, a way of accounting for the limitations of the medical paradigm to do what it claims it *can* do—explain illness through diagnosis—by transferring the responsibility for non-diagnosis to a cognitive domain.

Characterizing the absence of diagnosis as "uncertainty" uses indecision as its defense. To be uncertain is to negotiate between multiple options, to be in a position troubled by one, or many, other possibilities. But most importantly as a cognitive state, it is located in the *mind* of the individual clinician. When we talk about diagnostic uncertainty, we position the problem as one of individual expertise rather than as one of the generic diagnostic structure. Locating the problem of non-diagnosis in the individual clinician protects the paradigm.

In his work on the professions and the division of expert labor, Abbot (1988) attributes significant power to classifications systems. They are, he explains, how a profession maps its jurisdiction. Diagnosis is the means by which knowledge is adjudicated in medicine, and it is via its diagnostic framework that medicine has gained the authority "to define the real" (Whooley and Horwitz 2013, 20). When its diagnostic methods are insufficient to explain disease, it must still justify that diagnosis is an achievable aim.

Splitting from Diagnosis?

In 1927, William Stanley Sykes explained how important it was for patients to have a name for their disorders. It was a paradox, however, because a "bad" name, say a tumor, would be so soul destroying. "It is wiser and kinder to withhold the news as long as possible," he wrote (59). At the same time, he underlined the semiautomatic (yet mistaken) association of "tumor" with "cancer." Tumors aside, "Latinise a symptom and they'll feel safe," he continued (60).

Undeland and Malterud (2002) maintain that we err by seeing diagnosis as the be-all and end-all of the medical consultation. The encounter could be recast as a help-seeking interaction in which serious matters are diagnosed and symptoms managed, with reassignment, perhaps when matters brought to the doctor's attention belong in a category of care outside of the doctor's expertise, as described above. This is a particularly important point if, as Stone and colleagues suggest, "some diagnostic labels, particularly those that sound 'psychological,' can be perceived by patients as offensive by implying that the patients are 'putting on' or 'imagining' their symptoms or that they are 'mad.'"

Stone and his colleagues (2002) go further to explain that many diagnostic labels have a great ability to offend patients so labeled. They write that "although 'medically unexplained' is scientifically neutral, it had surprisingly negative connotations for patients." I do not find this surprising, because, as I have demonstrated above, although the label is neutral, its use is anything but. Stone calls for the restoration of the term "functional," which, despite suggesting a mental problem, appears to be acceptable to patients. The functional disorder provides "a rationale for pharmacological, behavioral, and psychological treatments aimed at restoring normal functioning . . . a useful and acceptable diagnosis for physical symptoms unexplained by disease" (Stone et al. 2002).

At one level, diagnosis can only be collective, because it is a classificatory tool, and classification is precisely about collecting. A diagnosis serves to label that which is the same in those who are dissimilar. This is the challenge of Ockham and the paradox of diagnosis. A disease label necessarily effaces some individual difference: a point that the suffering individual will know better than anyone else.

CHAPTER FIVE

Engines of Diagnosis

> It is a most extraordinary thing, but I never read a patent medicine
> advertisement without being impelled to the conclusion that I am
> suffering from the particular disease therein dealt with in its most
> virulent form.   JEROME K. JEROME (1889)

I have borrowed the term "engines" from Peter Conrad, who in his 2005 article in the *Journal of Health and Social Behavior* chose "engines of medicalization" to describe those new driving forces expanding the scope of medicine and medical authority. "Medicalization" is one of only a few sociological terms that has managed to integrate itself into popular and medical parlance (Furedi 2006). This process by which medical authority or explanations infiltrate banal social experiences of everyday life has infused scholarly literature since the early 1970s (Zola, Conrad, and Schneider are among the seminal writers in this area). Conrad argued that while early studies of the phenomenon tended to see medical imperialism at its root, in the contemporary context a number of new players are invested in promoting medical explanations for a range of conditions. Conrad's engines of medicalization emerge from the changing organization of health care, where biotechnology, consumers, and managed care organizations have elbowed in on the medical profession and social movements.

Medicalization is frequently, although not invariably, enabled by diagnostic categories. The demand for, or proposal of, a diagnosis may be the first step in casting life's experiences as medical. It is with this thought in mind that analysis of diagnosis becomes a useful activity. The fact that there is a diagnosis for this or that condition validates the fact that medical attention is warranted, a treatment justified, and an identity consolidated. It positions the condition in the medical arena and starts the ball rolling.

Disease labeling is but one of the many ways by which medicalization takes place. Further, the classification of a disease plays a substantive role outside of identifying recognized sickness: defining deviance, disciplining practitioners, setting research agendas, and distributing resources (Rosenberg 2002). And diagnoses hide both agendas and ideologies.

In this chapter, as Peter Conrad has done in relation to medicalization, I review a number of drivers of diagnosis, explicating the range of interests that can be served by the presence or awareness of particular disease entities. I then provide a case study of one particular diagnosis to demonstrate how it has become a focal point for a number of interests. The genesis, screening and treatment of female hypoactive sexual desire disorder (FHSDD) suggest the influence of powerful stakeholders and androcentric, heteronormative definitions of sexuality. It is not that female sexuality has not already been studied within the context of medicalization (see, for example, Tiefer 1996). This case study serves as a useful heuristic for understanding how classificatory systems describe "realities" that merit further critical scrutiny and how engines of diagnosis promote their existence.

I explore the layers of meaning embodied in the diagnosis of FHSDD, using some of the social framing mechanisms that Aronowitz (2008) has identified. Starting with the sociocultural framing of sexuality, particularly female sexuality, I demonstrate how fascination with the presumption of an immutable normative sexuality is unchallenged and untested in medicine. I then discuss the development of screening tools for the disease, which I present as technological mechanisms for reinforcing the presence of the diagnosis. And finally, I discuss the internal and external dynamics of consumption that constitute FHSDD as a diagnostic category. The prevalent use of the hypersexualized woman in all forms of media presents a fantasy of constant desire and sexual fulfillment and underlines the inadequacy of the consumer. A consumer solution is promoted by the pharmaceutical industry in the exercise of disease branding: marketing the diagnosis to create demand for its cure.

Engines of Diagnosis

Because, as we have discussed at length in previous chapters, disease classification is a social activity—fluid and contingent, and reliant upon knowledge, values, and social priorities—conditions become diseases at particular moments and in particular contexts. While medicine retains the ultimate authority for naming disease, there are a number of other drivers of disease labeling that we need to acknowledge.

In 1992, Payer introduced the term "disease monger" and identified a medical-industrial complex, which, she argued, has a significant interest in promoting the notion that the greater population is either already sick or at risk of becoming so. Her focus was on the abuse of diagnosis as a mechanism for advancing political, social, and commercial interests. She identified a range of agents that stood to benefit from the proliferation of diagnostic labels—creating a need for their products and services—including medical researchers, medical writers, health educators/promoters, the pharmaceutical and diagnostics industry, doctors, lawyers, hospitals, the courts, and insurance companies.

There has since been wide-ranging critical discussion of the clinical and economic contexts of disease mongering (Dear and Webb 2007; Healy 2006; Moncrieff, Hopker, and Thomas 2005; Moynihan and Cassels 2005; Moynihan, Heath, and Henry 2002; Payer 1992; Tiefer 2006; Wolinsky 2005), with an array of definitions. Payer (1992) describes mongering as "big business trying to convince essentially well people that they are sick, or slightly sick people that they are very ill." Moynihan, Heath, and Henry refer to "widening the boundaries of treatable illness in order to expand markets for those who sell and deliver treatments" (2002). Sociologists may have been slow to start focusing on the pharmaceutical industry, in great part owing to the discipline's focus on the experience of illness and inadequate scientific-technical knowledge and to the industry's secretiveness and the threat of legal challenge (Abraham 2007; Busfield 2006).

From within a sociology of diagnosis, however, it is useful to explore and, indeed, theorize about the phenomenon referred to by its critics as disease mongering, as diagnostic labels are at the fulcrum of its activities. To understand how diagnoses are promoted by nonmedical sources requires reflection that includes but goes beyond the pharmaceutical industry, and notably includes other industries as well as the context in which diagnosis currently takes place.

Let us not forget, either, the benefits that medicine itself stands to gain by promoting diagnosis. As I discuss throughout, it is a powerful thing to be able to label disease. Claiming diagnosis as within medicine's purview alone makes diagnostic power more elusive and more attractive. It is therefore not surprising that there will be tussles over it. A lot of players want a part of diagnosis, from the patient to other health care professions and biomedical industries. In a sense, by emphasizing the uniqueness and importance of diagnosis to its practice, medicine sets up a context in which others will try to insert their own interests.

The ability to promote diagnoses is facilitated by the diffusion of informational knowledge through e-scaped medicine, as described by Nettleton in chapter 3. In this context, control over medical information shifts from the doctor to a variety of other loci, with manifold motivations (in the case of industry, commercial). The patient becomes a "consumer," but not only in the commercial sense. A proliferation of information and media sites are available for ingestion: direct-to-consumer advertising, online self-screening tests, patient advocacy organizations, and disease awareness campaigns. Many of them are covertly, if not overtly, propped up by the industry, which stands to gain from expanding the number of individuals under a particular diagnostic umbrella.

Commercial interests have an important stake in highlighting overweight as a medical diagnosis, rather than a statistical deviation from normative weight. These interests go beyond the pharmaceutical industry. Fitness centers—part of a $30.6 billion industry in the United States in 2022 (Gough 2023)—in addition to the pharmaceutical and weight-loss industries and even some practicing physicians, rely heavily on promoting public belief in overweight-as-disease. Identifying obesity as a disease against which gym-goers can battle, reminding them of the ever-present "threat" of disease with body mass index charts, scales for self-monitoring, and doomsday publications about the risks of corpulence are important marketing tools—both of the diagnosis of obesity and of vigilant exercise, the first justifying the second.

A large number of industries stand to benefit from the belief that overweight is a disease. This results in significant lobbying and product promotion based on the disease label (Oliver 2006). Weight reduction, muscle tone, and body shape are exceptionally strong markers of "health" to consumers (Spitzack 1990). The gym, diet, self-help, cosmetic, pharmaceutical, fashion, publishing, and many other industries all have a financial stake in ensuring that people see their weight as problematic from a medical point of view (Jutel and Buetow 2007).

As Campos et al. (2006) have pointed out, even leading researchers in obesity (including those who set the criteria to determine what constitutes obesity) have an economic interest in defining overweight as widely as possible, either through their partnership with the pharmaceutical industry or their own private weight-loss clinics. Their preoccupation with overweight as disease defies evidence of lower mortality associated with overweight (BMI 25–29) than with normal weight (BMI 18.5–24.9) (Romero-Corral et al. 2006), health benefits of subcutaneous fat on hips and thighs (Nevill et al. 2006), and an increase in non-cancer mortality after weight loss (Nilsson et al. 2002).

Commercial influences are not the only nonmedical forces with an interest in promoting particular diagnoses. I have used the example of "excited delirium" previously in the text. One can well imagine what interests might be protected by the presence of this particular diagnosis. Even though the criteria for such "deliria" are far from established (Milliken 1998), attributing these unexpected deaths to disease rather than to excessive force fits comfortably with the presumed ethical behavior of the police or (in cases of restraint of the mentally ill) of care providers.

There are yet others with an incentive to promote particular diagnoses. Research teams, normally with—but sometimes without—commercial funding, are built around both legitimate and contested diseases. They attract private and public money to their institutions, together with students and high-profile staff (Burgan 2005). Similarly, politicians are often willing to engage in disease awareness campaigns to identify with and exploit popular concerns. For example, previous political campaigns in New Zealand used promises around screening for prostate disease and increased disease awareness as part of their election campaign strategy (Ryall 2007), despite recommendations from the New Zealand Guidelines Group that, even with the best possible estimates of the accuracy of the available screening tests, evidence does not support population-based screening for prostate cancer (Durham 2002).

The social media environment provides powerful leverage for all kinds of diagnostic engines, from mobile apps to diagnosis "pages," social advocacy groups, commercial promotion and self-diagnosis. As discussed in chapter 4, the use of nonmedical information, from Google to newspaper articles and every form of media in between, is not completely new; however, the proliferation of potential avenues via which the sick person can explore their disorder makes the effect strong.

The vast array of self-diagnosis and disease awareness tools that feature on Facebook pages, Twitter feeds, and health care digital apps are, more often than not, imbricated in usually hidden or partially obscured commercial endeavors. They serve to endorse tools, treatments, or technologies linked to the diagnoses they promote. The social importance of diagnosis is enhanced by technology and consumerism that takes advantage of the popular interest in disease categories in a circular relationship where the social importance is further reinforced by the hidden marketing to the digitally engaged patient-in-waiting (Lupton and Jutel 2015).

For the balance of this chapter, I discuss one particular diagnosis, FHSDD, whose promotion is firmly driven by a range of commercial, medical, and pharmaceutical interests. It serves, I hope, as a poignant example of exactly what Jerome K. Jerome describes, perhaps humorously, as his own reaction to patent medicine advertisements. The importance of diagnostic recognition is a valuable tool for those whose interests reside in public health (it *is* good to be able to recognize influenza, malaria, and chronic urinary tract infections) but also for those whose interests reside in commercial gain.

Leonore Tiefer (2006) argues that the creation and promotion of a diagnosis of "female sexual dysfunction" was influenced by a convergence of three factors: pharmaceutical companies, urologists closely associated with this industry, and media-savvy sex therapists operating in the for-profit sector. The acute interest in women's sexuality, she maintains, is linked to uncritical definitions of what constitutes normal female sexuality. It is also part of the industry's desire to expand the market for drugs like Viagra by promoting erectile dysfunction more widely than is justified (Lexchin 2006).

Female Hypoactive Sexual Desire Disorder

The matter of female libido, or at least of the association of gender with libido, is one which has preoccupied scholars for centuries. While a historical survey is beyond the scope of this chapter, a bouquet of examples from various eras can still illustrate this fascination.

The oft-cited myth of Tiresias, as recounted by Ovid, is a useful starting point. Tiresias was called upon by the gods Jupiter and Juno to settle their argument about whether the sexual pleasure of man or woman was greatest. He was appointed to "arbitrate this jocular dispute" because he had "known both Venuses" (Ovid 1985, 105), having lived seven years as a woman after having been born a man. He agreed with Jupiter: women have more pleasure. Tiresias's decision was not without consequence. Juno blinded him for his taking Jupiter's side. To palliate his loss of sight, Jupiter gave him the ability to know the future (Ovid 1985).

While medieval writers sought to demonstrate that the organs and orgasms of men and women reflected one another, the pudenda responding like the penis during coitus, Renaissance doctors struggled to make physiological sense of female orgasm. Women were variably cast as passionless or as insatiable libidinal beasts. These polar attitudes filled medical and philosophical texts. Concern about sexual difference served as a proxy for anxiety about power and position in the public sphere (Laqueur 1990).

In Victorian times, medicine, concerned about sexual excesses, took responsibility for education about sexuality, seeking both to explain and modulate the place of desire in woman's social role and to link it with the production of healthy offspring. Some authors argued that female passion had a physiological link to conception, a position George Napheys (1871) refuted in his late nineteenth-century guidebook for women. He argued, nonetheless, that the "disposition" of the woman at the time of conception had a formative effect on the physical and emotional formation of the fetus and described three levels of sexuality in women. There are those who have generally little or no sexual feeling, he wrote, a second group, probably slightly greater than the previous, who are "more or less subject to strong passion," and finally the "vast majority of women in whom the sexual appetite is as moderate as all other appetites" (74).

Another popular medical writer, Frederick Hollick, acknowledged a wide difference between the two sexes "as to the manner in which the imagination acts, owing to the difference in their characters and organization" (1902, 395). He maintained that a woman, in addition to her desire to please, also has an innate sentiment of *shame*, which can lead to prudery if dominant. But he also cautioned that when "the [woman's] temperament is warm, and the sexual instinct unusually strong . . . indulgence is imperatively needed, and if it cannot be had the most injurious consequences may take place, indicating the possibility of miscarriage and partial derangement" (389). Physician Mary Ries Melendy (1904), meanwhile, cautioned that in the sexual union, the wife should "not be overtaxed beyond her natural desire" should the couple be in pursuit of a high spiritual life (310).

Although medical guides and handbooks addressed the matter of female sexual desire, pathologization of low libido became part of the nomenclature only in the last quarter of the twentieth century. At the beginning of that century, medicine was preoccupied with *excessive* female desire (Lunbeck 1987). It was not until 1980 that the *DSM-III* (Rogler 1997) introduced a diagnosis of "inhibited sexual desire," a condition reported as more common in women and described as the "persistent and pervasive inhibition of sexual desire. The judgment of inhibition is made by the clinician's taking into account factors that affect sexual desire such as age, sex, health, intensity and frequency of sexual desire, and the context of the individual's life. In actual practice this diagnosis will rarely be made unless the lack of desire is a source of distress to either the individual or his or her partner" (278). In 1987, the *DSM-III-R* recast the diagnosis as "hypoactive sexual desire disorder," described now as "persistently or recurrently deficient or absent sexual fantasies and desire for sexual activity. The judgment of deficiency or absence is made by the clinician, taking into account factors that affect sexual functioning, such as age, sex, and the context of the person's life" (293). The integration of these classifications into the *International Classification of Diseases* was made somewhat later. "Inhibited sexual desire" may have figured in the 1977 *ICD-9*, but "hypoactive sexual desire" was not present until the *ICD-10* (1993).

The diagnosis of FHSDD relies on the untested assumption that all humans are endowed with demonstrable sexual urges and that their absence constitutes a pathological condition. This constitutes the fundamental structural frame to buttress the pathologization of low or non-existent sexual desire. Masters and Johnson presented sexuality as "a drive of biologic origin deeply integrated into the condition of human existence," an important cornerstone, argues Tiefer (1996), to the development of alleged universal, biological sexual norms.

A facile evolutional argument supporting this assumption is that sexual urges are a biological necessity for the survival of the species. I use the word "facile" advisedly. That same-sex sexuality challenges this assumption is the easiest rejoinder. While homosexuality continues to present collective challenges to a heterosexually dominant classificatory society, its nonreproductive sexual urges are no longer contained in the *DSM*, enunciating clearly that evolution doesn't determine what medicine chooses to classify.

As a result of this presumption, there has been little contemporary scholarly discussion of asexuality in other-than-medical terms. Being captured by medicine defuses threats to any social assumptions; medicine becomes simultaneously the explanation and the discipliner. Its classificatory status announces this is "the way things are" and thwarts challenges.

Kaplan (1977) is cited (in Sills et al. 2005) as one of the earliest contemporary medical researchers to discuss low sexual urge in terms of pathology, building on the interest in sexuality promoted by the work of Masters and Johnson. While she acknowledged that there is no definition of normal sexual urge, she pointed out that the sex therapy literature failed to address matters of sexual desire. She presented low urge as a problem requiring extensive therapy and associated it with a fear of love, success, and pleasure. In the same year, Lief (1977) reported that inhibited sexual desire affected 37 percent of women in one sample and was among the most difficult sexual dysfunctions to treat. Kaplan's and Lief's interest in the issue of sexual desire as an area of therapeutic interest was enabled by the sexual liberation movement of the previous decade and its breaking down of sexual taboos.

More recent medical work tends to be epidemiological, confirming prevalence, incidence, and associations (always, however, emphasizing asexuality-as-pathology by confirming FSHDD as something worthy of counting). Bogaert (2004)—on the basis of preexisting data from the UK National Survey of Sexual Attitudes and Lifestyles—reports that 1 percent of the population claimed to have no sexual attraction to members of either sex. He identifies a number of associated and predictive features of asexuality, including gender (mainly women), religiosity, short stature, low education, low socioeconomic status, and poor health.

In contradistinction to this epidemiological approach to understanding asexuality, identity-based discussions take a different tack. A number of internet communities have sprung up for individuals who identify as asexual. Virtual communities in a general sense provide a sanctuary for alternative and stigmatized groups. Notable for their genesis in medical-lay discord about diagnosis, these groups may provide support for illnesses that medicine does not sanction (for example, see Dumit [2006] on medically unexplained symptoms; Ware [1992] on chronic fatigue; or Charland [2004] on psychiatric disorders). Or a site might reject a medically imposed diagnostic classification, seeking to redefine what medicine perceives as disease in other terms (for example, see Fox, Ward, and O'Rourke's work on the pro-anorexia movement [2005]; or St-Onge, Provencher, and Ouellet on psychosis [2005]).

Scherrer (2008) studied participants in the Asexual Visibility and Education Network and concluded, among other things, that the language to define and the space to be asexual offered by the virtual community enabled individuals to construct an essential identity based on the absence of sexual drive. She also suggested that asexuality has had far less attention paid to it than other sexual identities. Possibly as a result of its *lack* of behavior and desire, it does not draw attraction to itself and has not historically been perceived as morally or legally wrong (Bogaert 2004). Her respondents, for the most part, saw asexuality as aproblematic and naturalized it as a way of being, rather than as an ontological illness.

Prause and Graham (2007) surveyed the sexuality of 1,146 students and found 41 who identified as asexual. Of these, 63.4 percent (n = 26) were women. These men and women attributed both benefits and drawbacks to asexuality. Benefits included avoiding intimate relationship problems, having lower health risks and social pressures, and having more free time. Drawbacks were potential partner relationship problems, thinking something is wrong, negative public perception, and missing positive aspects of sex. Prause and Graham also write that asexual individuals may feel pressure to conform to the normative expectation of sexuality, a social expectation that goes beyond the control of the individual. The existence of the diagnostic category, more than the lack of sexual drive itself, however, may provide a shove toward the illness. Because personal distress is a diagnostic criterion for FHSDD, and because distress results from worry that asexuality may be a medical problem, "then the psychiatric diagnosis implying abnormality may exacerbate concerns in an asexual individual" (353).

Social theory provides a perspective that challenges the pathologization of low sexual drive. In both queer and feminist theory, gender and sexuality are cast as products of social and historical context rather than of immutable biological states. Trends in social theory conceptualize these categories as plural, provisional, and situated (D. Richardson 2007), providing space for asexuality as a normal form of sexuality.

The "Boston marriage," or romantic but asexual lesbian relationship, has a long historical, albeit unacknowledged, tradition (Rothblum and Brehony 1993). Boston marriages challenge the idea that sexual activity defines relationships. Women in such relationships may or may not previously have had sexual relations between themselves or with others but no longer do so. In all other ways, their relationship resembles those of other lesbian couples. Importantly though, the fact of their asexuality is neither acknowledged nor broadcast. To do so would be both a political and social liability.

Naomi McCormick (in Rothblum and Brehony 1993) sees the demand for sexual pleasure as proxy for partnership as a reflection of an androcentric approach to sexuality: "It is entirely possible that many passionate female friendships enjoyed by our foremothers excluded mutual genital stimulation that people expect before categorizing a relationship as sexual or erotic. The absence of genital juxtaposition hardly drains a relationship of passion or importance" (6). Jagose (2003) echoes McCormick's comments: "That such happy, well-matched couples can be so easily drawn into the jurisdiction of pathological dysfunction suggests something of the weird morphing effect of the medical/therapeutic industries on the cultural status or value of sexual desire. Not in itself necessarily desirable, desire is instead compulsory. It turns out to be banally more like the Brussels sprouts of childhood, something that is good for us and that we must have whether we like it or not."

This contextualization is muted in the assumptions underpinning the diagnosis of FHSDD. That hyposexuality is seen to be a medical problem further reinforces the taboos around discussing love without sex. Rothblum and Brehony (1993) point out that many members of the lesbian community kept their asexuality hidden, because being "out" as lesbians required them to be a model of normative lesbian relationships.

The diagnosis of FHSDD, however, disregards the historical and social context of sexuality; rather, it focuses on clinical detail about attitudes toward sex. The tools of diagnosis constitute a second important framing mechanism in creating the classification itself.

Technological Change

There is a technology of FHSDD that is generative. As with the diagnosis of overweight (discussed in chapter 2), FHSDD cannot establish an epidemiological existence in the absence of a mechanism for assessing its presence. Powerful interests, I argue, are at play in the rush to develop the tools to establish the existence of FHSDD. Not the least of these are on the panel of the "International Consensus Development Conference on Female Sexual Dysfunction," whose authoritative professional status elevates its recommendations to the status of mandates. The preliminary meetings to develop the consensus conference were organized by the industry and were made up of a group intentionally balanced between pharmaceutical representatives and researchers either experienced or interested in working collaboratively with the industry (Moynihan 2003).

This group identified the penury of studies investigating female sexual dysfunction and the barrier presented by the absence of diagnostic frameworks (Basson et al. 2000). This call to action was supported by grants from Eli Lilly, Pentech, Pfizer, Procter & Gamble, Schering-Plough, Solway Pharmaceuticals, TAP Pharmaceuticals, and Zonagen, just as its 19 authors acknowledged financial or other relationships with 24 listed pharmaceutical companies. The findings of this committee were that urgent investigation was required to develop new classifications and definitions of sexual dysfunction.

The first specific instrument for assessing FHSDD or its response to various treatments was developed by Sills and colleagues and presented in 2005. Titled the validated Sexual Interest and Desire Inventory–Female (SIDI-F), the work was both funded and copyrighted by the pharmaceutical company Boehringer Ingelheim and undertaken by its scientists (Sills et al. 2005). I detail overleaf Boehringer Ingelheim's interest in FHSDD. Sills and his colleagues tested the 17-item rating scale on women previously diagnosed by an experienced clinician as having FHSDD. His pilot study tested the tool on 21 participants, 9 without the disorder and 12 with. He concludes that the scale could be used to discriminate between participants diagnosed with FHSDD and those without a clinical diagnosis, but he does not provide data from the pilot. The main study tests only women with the disorder, failing to validate sensitivity in a second independent group of patients, thus limiting the predictive value of the instrument.

A recent publication, however, purports to supersede the SIDI-F. It is a streamlined survey tool that, its authors argue, enables nonspecialists to deal with the fraught problem of female sexual function. They describe a "growing need for simple diagnostic instruments that can be used in everyday practice by clinicians who are not specialists or experts in FSD" (Clayton et al. 2009, 731).

The Decreased Sexual Desire Screener (DSDS) (Clayton et al. 2009) is designed by its researchers to provide a very brief tool that can be used by nonspecialists to diagnose what the authors believe is a very prevalent condition among women. The tool has two parts. The woman is presented with an initial set of four questions. If she answers all of them *affirmatively*, then she will answer a second set of questions. If she answers all of these *negatively*, the clinician can confirm the diagnosis of FHSDD. The simplicity of the diagnostic

procedure is beguiling, but both the nature of the questions and the relationship of the researchers to the commercial players in the sexual dysfunction
industry give pause. The first four questions ask:

1. In the past, was your level of sexual desire/interest good and satisfying to you?
2. Has there been a decrease in your level of sexual desire/interest?
3. Are you bothered by your decreased level of sexual desire/interest?
4. Would you like your level of sexual desire/interest to increase?

A fifth question rules out other causes for the decreased sexual interest (relationship problems, systemic illness, recent obstetric or gynecological events,
stress, or fatigue).

Nonspecialist clinicians in the field of female sexual dysfunction then reviewed the responses and determined whether the individuals met the criteria
for generalized, acquired FHSDD. Subsequently, expert clinicians conducted a
standard diagnostic interview with each participant. Results of the interview
and those of the DSDS were then compared to validate the diagnostic ability
of the tool. Yet both the predictive value of this tool and the interests of the
researcher who developed it must be questioned.

Predictive value reflects the probability that the tool will correctly and predictably identify the presence of the condition. This means that its use will not
wrongly identify individuals without the disorder as having it. Intuitively, one
senses that the four questions that comprise the DSDS are most likely to result
in an affirmative response from many women and that the confirming set of
questions will also result in a likely negative response, which would result in
a positive diagnosis. The fact that the study was validated in a population with
a high prevalence of the disorder limits its ability to project across a general
population.

The interests of the researcher are also important to describe. Anita Clayton is a consultant for Boehringer Ingelheim, whose relationship to FHSDD I
discuss in greater depth in the next section. There I explore the dynamics of
consumption, including the commodification of sexuality by pharmaceutical
companies such as Boehringer Ingelheim.

Commodity Culture

On the topic of the dynamics of consumption, Aronowitz describes how
the effective manipulation of consumer need negatively affects physical and
mental health, resulting in identification of a problem as medical. In the case

of female sexuality, the commercial dynamic is twofold. It presents the sexual woman both as commodity and as consumer. This dual burden of consumer longing and disease classification is not unprecedented. The nineteenth-century disease of kleptomania typified women as simultaneously consumers of, and consumed by, shopping (Roberts 1998).

FHSDD reflects this two-way street of commodity culture, in which longing for spontaneous hypersexuality is marketed, then pathologized and re-presented with its concomitant cure similarly available as a consumer item. The pharmaceutical industry acts as "an engine of medicalization" (P. Conrad 2005), transforming longing into disease. Classification (diagnosis) confirms the presumed ontological, always-already-there illness.

FHSDD's presence in commodity culture is anchored in the sale of sexuality and the public discourse that surrounds female hypersexuality in product sales. From music videos to milk advertisements, the sexually provocative display of the female body in enticingly erotic postures is common currency (Reichert and Lambiase 2003). This positions hypersexuality as a female norm. Women are supposed to like having sex and being sexy. Not wanting sex is not normal. So, the readers of *Woman's Weekly* and *Woman's Day* follow the thousand little rules for achieving a bikini body in time for summer, simultaneously taking surveys about what turns them on, how to make *him* (not her) happy in bed, and figuring out just how often they should be having sex (if they're normal, that is) and of what kind. The vexed question of "just how often are normal people having sex?" surfaces in publications from *Glamour* to *New Scientist* and figures in self-screening tools about longevity, happiness, and relationship health.

This might be the pursuit of what Cushman argues is a great consumer yearning, emerging from the transformation of the bounded, restricted Victorian self into the empty post–World War II self-contained individual. This "empty self" finds its fulfillment in consumption and acquisition, with sexuality a prevalent theme. Glorified sexual images whose primary intent is to sell products present at the same time a mandate to be sexy, to have sex, and to desire sexual connection (Kilbourne 2003).

Sex sells magazines, clothes, cosmetics, cars, music, toothpaste, and a myriad of other items, but the reciprocal is also true: magazines, clothes, cosmetics, cars, music, and toothpaste sell sex. The fantasy of constant desire and sexual fulfillment captured in advertising serves as a perpetual punctuation of the inadequacy of the consumer (Kilbourne 2003). It is a distortion of reality, presenting sexuality as it should be (at least in the eyes of able marketers), not as it is. The consumer then seeks to attain normality as it is portrayed in the imaginary. The transformation of longing into pathology is being skillfully managed by a number of players in the pharmaceutical industry, creating a second tier in the commercial dynamic that generates FHSDD as a diagnostic category (Tiefer 2006).

The story of FHSDD infused by the efforts of the pharmaceutical industry to establish the existence of female sexual dysfunction in order to market the cure. But we'll start with the cure, to understand where the stakes are driven and how the commercial interest is promoted. The story hinges around the medication flibanserin, patented in 2006 as a treatment for FSHDD (Borsini and Evans 2006).

The primary component of flibanserin, a compound called BIMT 17, was initially investigated as a potential antidepressant, appearing in the psychopharmacology literature for the first time in 1997 (Borsini et al. 1997) after animal studies two years earlier (Borsini et al. 1995). The first author of these articles is a staff scientist for Boehringer Ingelheim. His work describes the substance as having a faster possible onset of therapeutic action than other established therapeutic options for depression. Later media reports about the compound reveal that during early phase studies of its antidepressant activity, researchers monitored anticipated side effects of decreased libido and observed, rather than the expected decrease, an increase (Carey 2006). There is no published research heralding this finding. But by December 2006, Borsini and a colleague from Canada had filed a US patent application on behalf of Boehringer Ingelheim for a "method of treating female hypoactive sexual desire disorder with Flibanserin" (Borsini and Evans 2006).

Boehringer Ingelheim (BI) launched a media campaign proclaiming the importance of flibanserin and the severity of FHSDD. On October 31, 2008, BI released a press release touting that "the largest study of its kind reveals low sexual desire is [the] most common female sexual problem" (Meyer-Kleinmann 2008a), citing Shifren and colleagues' (2008) cross-sectional survey of 31,581 female respondents that reported 38.7 percent of women experienced low desire. The science behind the findings seems clear. The sample size is exceptional, the p values and confidence intervals stringent, the scale used to determine FHSDD validated.

Closer scrutiny reveals, however, that the study was funded by Boehringer Ingelheim, that the principle author on this paper receives consulting fees from BI, that the second and third authors were employed by BI at the time of the research, and that the remaining authors "performed work related to this article under a research contract with BI and their employer" (Shifren et al. 2008). The scale used to validate the condition was developed outside of BI, but by researchers funded by a different pharmaceutical industry player, Procter & Gamble (Derogatis et al. 2002). Procter & Gamble had a similar interest in promoting female sexual distress, given its commitment to Intrinsa, a transdermal testosterone patch for the treatment of FHSDD (Drug and Therapeutics Bulletin 2009).

Buttressed by science generated by the pharmaceutical industry itself, Boehringer Ingelheim set forth on an awareness campaign to highlight the frequency, underdiagnosis, and consequences of FHSDD (see Meyer-Kleinmann's [2008b] press release). The company prepared an information sheet describing an unreferenced frequency of "up to one in five women" and promoting a new diagnostic tool comprising only five questions, taking less than 15 minutes (BI 2008). This is the DSDS referred to above, developed and validated by Anita Clayton and her team. As I have pointed out, Clayton is a consultant to, is funded by, and is on the advisory board of Boehringer Ingelheim. Her article reporting on the validation of the DSDS was not published until March 2009 in the *Journal of Sexual Medicine*. BI's announcement preceded the publication of the actual study. The *Journal of Sexual Medicine*, however, was an ally of the pharmaceutical industry whose websites historically featured professional endorsements from various pharmaceutical companies.

Of course, Clayton is not the only researcher in this area with strong ties to industry. The medical opinion leaders in the discussion of FHSDD are, for the most part, affiliated with Boehringer Ingelheim or with related industry players. From the consensus writers in 1999, who originally set the scene, to the authors of recent reviews of the condition and the expert clinicians developing tools, most have an affiliation with Boehringer Ingelheim either through funding of the studies being reported or in a consultant role (Clayton et al. 2009; Shifren et al. 2008; Sills et al. 2005; and so on). Boehringer Ingelheim is not alone in funding the tools and providing cures for female sexual dysfunction. I have previously mentioned Procter & Gamble, but Pfizer (and perhaps others) also has a vested interest in the development of other treatments for female sexual dysfunction.

Since the first edition of this book was published, the FDA gave flibanserin the nod, despite reports of ineffectiveness and safety concerns. A small added safety study on interactions with alcohol presented in 2015 was poorly designed (a sample of 25 participants including only two women) and showed results that were less than reassuring. When used with alcohol, flibanserin caused such large drops in blood pressure in one-fourth of participants that they required medical intervention (FDA 2015). The most likely reason for flibanserin's approval was intense pressure on the FDA through the "Even the Score" campaign, which characterized the FDA's refusal to approve the drug as sexist, arguing that men had many drug treatments for sexual problems and women had none (Gellad et al. 2015; Woloshin and Schwartz 2016).

Flibanserin was approved over the objection of the FDA's clinical reviewers and cross-disciplinary team leader (FDA 2015; Woloshin and Schwartz 2016). The main rationale provided by the FDA was that "there are no approved medications for HSDD, that the condition can cause substantial distress and have profound effects on relationships and well-being, that some women have a clinically meaningful response to treatment" (Joffe 2015). The FDA stated that around 10 percent more women taking the 100-milligram-per-day dose than those on placebo had a meaningful benefit (FDA 2015). The drug's frequent side effects of sleepiness, fatigue, dizziness, and nausea, however, would have meant that many women in the study likely guessed correctly they were on the drug (Jaspers et al. 2016).

Ironically, the most problematic outcome in all of the flibanserin trials was the one that the drug aims to treat: desire. The first three trials were designed to have a combined primary outcome measure of the number of satisfying sexual events that a woman had in each 28-day period and keep a daily "e-diary" recordings of her sexual desire level. For the drug to be considered more effective than a placebo, it needed to do significantly better on both counts. The woman's e-diary asked her to record each day what her most intense level of sexual desire was, ranging from "no desire" to "strong desire." The stronger the recorded desire per day, the better a woman is assumed to be doing. In other words, the best score comes from a report of strong desire on all days. In all three studies, women's daily reports of their desire levels failed to differ significantly between drug and placebo (FDA 2015).

These results highlight both the odd definition of ideal sexuality in these trials and the elusiveness of efficacy measures when desire—a highly socially and culturally charged phenomenon—is the anticipated effect. Despite these conundrums, female hypoactive sexual desire disorder provides a powerful example of the fascination with female sexuality as a matter for medical concern. What the diagnosis has also managed to forge is considerable opposition. There is not space in this chapter to explore it in depth, but it should be noted that while the pharmaceutical industry has rather cynically used women's equality as a tool for its own purposes, its actions have generated considerable dissent. Organizations such as New View (http://www.newviewcampaign.org/) and Pharmed Out (http://www.pharmedout.org/) have taken powerful stances to counter the arguments that (1) low sexual urge should be seen as problematic and even when it is, that (2) doctors and medicines should be the preferred solution. Although the pursuit of pharmaceutical enhancement of women's libido looked to place low libido under medical control for the foreseeable future, time will tell whether it has in fact done the opposite.

The consumer dynamic is clearly complex. It involves an initial and pervasive representation to the consumer of sexuality as a means of escape from the real conditions of existence. Sexuality circulates as an attainable promise that must be eternally deferred for the promise to be unendingly remade (Brady 2007). On the one hand, consumer culture is based on perpetuating feelings of sexual inadequacy; on the other, the industry has recognized an opportunity for exploitation and has designed and presented a panacea, also for sale.

Discussion

Moving away, for a moment, from FHSDD, we should consider that this is neither the first nor the only way women's putative diseases reflect social understandings about the way women should be. Tacit cultural knowledge about the nature of women and of femininity is widely captured in the guise of objective, scientific fact. From the ancient Greeks, who claimed that hysteria was caused by a lack of sexual intercourse (Rodin 1992), to Victorians doctors, who maintained that a woman's menses prevented her from engaging in physical or intellectual activity (Vertinsky 1994), it has been common practice throughout the history of women's diseases to assert that symptoms are related to women's sexuality and conformity (or lack of) to prescribed social roles.

Premenstrual syndrome emerges from Hippocrates's hysteria, transformed along the way by the logic of *Malleus Maleficarum* (which held that women were prone to alliances with the devil) and by Renaissance thinkers who envisioned hysteria as a neurological disease. In 1931, the condition was first delineated in a formal, clinical context as "premenstrual tension." Emotional symptoms of premenstrual tension included nervousness, irritability, depression, and generalized emotional tension. "Premenstrual syndrome" was coined in 1953. Despite researchers' failure to scientifically link the stated emotional qualities to PMS, the connection has remained in medical discourse (Rodin 1992).

Diseases associated with the female menstrual cycle have a controversial recent history. The *DSM-III-R* included late luteal phase dysphoric disorder, or LLPDD, defined as a psychiatric disorder characterized by recurrent, cyclic periods of dysphoria corresponding with the menstrual cycle. Other physical and emotional symptoms associated with PMS were not included, and according to the *DSM-III-R*, only 5 percent of those with PMS would qualify as LLPDD.

Those in favor of including LLPDD in the *DSM* argued that it would stimulate research and encourage doctors to treat women's complaints more seriously. Opponents countered that women would be inappropriately diagnosed as mentally ill, or alternatively, women could use the diagnosis to justify criminal behavior (Rodin 1992). The Committee on Women of the American Psychiatric Association, with the help of professional and lay women's groups, argued that even a very carefully worded definition of the disease could be misconstrued so that all menstruating women could be dismissed as "crazy." Part of the debate centered on the nature of the disease. Hormonal disorders should be the purview of endocrinologists. But if it is mainly emotional, then it is rightfully managed by psychiatrists. Social workers and psychologists, on the contrary, claimed that it should be under their jurisdiction, since the problem was social and situational. Feminist social groups protested that it was a normal physiological process, and they pushed for self-treatment and alternative therapies. The Office of Research on Women's Health utilized feminist networks and the mailing list of the National Coalition for Women's Mental Health, encouraging a letter-writing campaign to the American Psychiatric Association. They were also able to focus media and the public's attention on the matter, delaying the publication of the *DSM-III-R* by two years (Lorber 1997).*

Perhaps an even more controversial women's diagnosis was the gendered self-depreciating personality disorder, originally to be called masochist per-

---

* A tentative diagnosis of LLPDD was placed in a special appendix titled "Proposed Diagnostic Categories Needing Further Study" in the *DSM-III-R*. In the *DSM-IV*, LLPDD was then renamed "premenstrual dysphoric disorder" and was still located in the appendix as a disputed disorder requiring further study (Busfield and Campling 1996). The *ICD-10* provides a code F32.81 for premenstrual dysphoric disorder. In the *DSM-5*, it is included under "depressive disorders" coded as 625.4.

sonality disorder (MPD). According to the draft for the *DSM-III-R*, women with MPD would make no demands on others, be self-sacrificing, experience discomfort with success and recognition, feel unworthy, and neglect their own pleasure for that of others (Kutchins and Kirk 1997). Feminist groups argued that MPD would be used to describe women who were in abusive relationships. The features of this proposed diagnosis have been lauded social characteristics of the ideal woman, creating paradoxically a disease out of heroic femininity. Literary examples of MPD sufferers would astound readers of women's fiction: Beth in *Little Women*, Melanie in *Gone with the Wind*, Sara in *The Little Princess*, and Mary in the *Little House* series were held as sainted examples of proper womanhood, as they were self-effacing, generous, unflinching, and probably—according to these diagnostic criteria—ill. The neoliberal context of self-interest, self-promotion, and individual self-realization does not celebrate these visions of femininity; rather, it promotes a discourse of freedom and flexibility.

This would be a case of what Gaines (1992) describes as the "voice of classification" valuing self-control and self-mastery, of privileging an ideal gender (male), ethnicity (German Protestant), and age (adult) over others. Because women do not fit into the idealized self, they are the focus of considerable attention in the *DSM*.

FHSDD is a vivid example of how the convergence of social circumstances leads first to the identification of a particular condition as problematic and second to its embodiment in a diagnostic framework. In this case, the disease category is relatively transparent but no less controlling. It would be simplistic to argue that FHSDD is simply the creation of the pharmaceutical industry, a perfect example of disease mongering. Without minimizing the role of the industry in the promotion and expansion of this diagnosis, I maintain that the industry cannot conjure a classification out of thin air.

A particular social context must provide the backdrop for the disease branding that Boehringer Ingelheim is undertaking with FHSDD. In this case, an age-old angst over women's sexuality overlaid by the commodification of sexuality provides a context within which the industry can drive for public and professional recognition of this disorder, rather than leaving it hidden in the pages of the *DSM* or the *ICD*, pulled out and dusted off for only the odd idiosyncratic case. In the case of FHSDD, the pharmaceutical industry alone could not make the diagnosis a wider concern if, for example, female sexuality was still generally taken as woman's duty to her spouse and nation. Imagine for a moment if those who counseled young married women today still believed J. A. Stewart's 1814 "advice previous to matrimony," that "the tumult of passion will necessarily subside" (540). The very first questions of Clayton's DSDS screening tool would, in that context, make no sense. Rather than capturing a picture of pathology, they would be describing the normal state of affairs: yes, my level of desire used to be good; yes, my level desire is lower than it was; yes, my passion has subsided.

While Stewart doesn't incriminate passion as deviant, by the turn of the next century, female hypersexuality figured large in psychiatric medicine as an ailment. Psychiatrists used the term "psychopathic" to describe women who engaged in sexual activity beyond the bounds of what genteel society considered moral (Lunbeck 1987). Such women were cast as sexual predators who sought to entrap young men through their "uncontrolled sex impulses," in stark contrast with the medical concern over female sexuality today.

For FHSDD to exist, sexuality must be a desired female attribute, and women capable of indulging their impulses without recrimination. Perpetual reminders of both factors serve to reposition the self as one who can have FHSDD. The transformation from the dangerous Victorian self, whose sexual and aggressive impulses had to be controlled by state and church, to the self-expressive, consuming, and indulgent self is an important prerequisite to any commercial strategy using inadequate sexuality as foundation (Cushman 1990). Cushman rightly maintains that understanding the configuration of the self and its temporal context provides insights on "the illnesses that plague it, and the activities responsible for healing it" (599).

Knowing what consumers feel and believe is an important foundation to any branding campaign, and Boehringer Ingelheim's intimate involvement in the promotion, identification, and cure of FHSDD is an exercise in disease branding. This approach markets not the therapy but rather the awareness of the condition that the therapy is supposed to cure. An effective disease-branding strategy results in sufficient public awareness such that intervention is no longer required: the patient and doctor are vigilant monitors of the potential for diagnosis (Parry 2007).

Understanding the diagnosis and its genesis provides another angle for understanding the medicalization of women's sexuality. First, the mechanisms that frame this diagnostic label, as described above, are firmly grounded in a social context that must be acknowledged. The diagnosis enables the expansion of medical authority and its agents (or "engines"). Second, the FHSDD label fulfills the potent social roles one expects of a diagnosis. It legitimizes deviance, defines normality, creates identity, and enables access to treatment (Jutel 2010a). Finally, however, it reinforces an inadequately challenged combination of assumptions and observations about sexual function that consequently serve as a basis for commercial exploitation and disease promotion.

CHAPTER SIX

Technologies of Diagnosis

Who is able by seeing the blood to divine whether it be an intermittent or a continuall feavor, whether a dysentery or haemoptoe the patient is sick of, and what sensible fault does often appear in that bloud in which nature does sometimes expel the cause of a disease, and give present ease by a critical haemorrhagia wherein the bloud very often looks as florid and as well conditioned as any that flows in the veins of the most healthy man living?   JOHN LOCKE (QTD. IN DEWHURST 1966)

John Locke was an empiricist and a skeptic. He firmly believed that medicine could advance only through experience and observation (Wolfe 1961). His medicine was typified by observed phenomena, external resemblances, and practical classification of diseases and their treatments. He maintained that the warrant of medicine was to save people from death, rather than to engage in the discovery of causes. In his view, looking for causes was a rather luxurious intellectual pursuit that did little to serve humanity. Locke considered this a form of speculation that did not aid practice. His objections to the study of the cause of disease may be grounded in the technological limitations of his era: "Nature performs all her operations on the body by parts so minute and insensible that I thinke noe body will ever hope or pretend, even by the assistance of glasses . . . , to come to a sight of them" (qtd. in Wolfe 1961, 213).

Locke's reluctance to use technology in medical research bears little resemblance to contemporary approaches to health and illness. Modern approaches highlight the powerful capacity of technology to contribute to the empirical: to perceive that which the naked eye—or the phenomenon-experiencing subject—cannot. We are accustomed to the blood test, the urine culture, or the X-ray to confirm "what we've got." We might even be suspicious of the clinician who delivers a diagnosis with minimal technological support, who draws on palpation, auscultation, patient account, or other clinical observations to arrive at a conclusion. "How do they know it's not something else?"

This is not the first time that technology has surfaced as an actor in diagnosis in the pages of this book. I have touched on the diagnostic role of technology in previous chapters. The introduction of classificatory categories (new diagnoses) is contingent upon technological advancement, just as the act of diagnosis may rely on and promote technology in preference to clinical observation and the patient's own report.

Technology is an important social force in diagnosis, shaping how we can understand disease categories and what categories we are not only able, but willing, to acknowledge. But technology is not neutral. This is not to say that it is not vital to the medicine and to overcoming illness—we'd be loath to return to an era of prescientific medicine—but it has social content, it trumps other forms of information, and its impact on the experience of disease is non-negligible.

Technology plays an increasingly important role in Western medicine. Since the mid-1980s, medicine has changed and extended its authority via an increasingly technoscientific formulation. Risk is monitored; medical knowledges are produced and consumed differently; information is standardized, quantified, scrutinized, and analyzed; identities are recreated along molecular and genetic lines (Clarke et al. 2003). Technology establishes, monitors, recognizes and treats diseases. In the following pages, I examine some of the ways technology fulfills these tasks.

Technology and Diagnostic Categories

As was the case with Alzheimer disease and the discovery of neurofibrillary tangles that I discussed in chapter 4, technology is often at the base of what medicine is capable of defining as illness. Recall that it was advanced staining techniques that enabled Alzheimer to distinguish this particular form of cognitive decline from the more mundane senility of old age. Technological advances enable the recognition of many other diagnostic categories. In sickle-cell anemia, for example, diagnostic labeling could never have taken place without the ability to create a laboratory profile of human blood, viewing sickle-shaped red blood cells on glass slides. The disease itself presented with varying clinical pictures but was not clearly distinguishable from other anemias, parasitic ailments, and syphilis. It was the microscopic profile of the "sickling" cell that enabled the creation of a new diagnosis. The blood smear, more than the clinical presentation, was at the heart of this diagnosis, coined in 1922 by Verne Mason (Feldman and Tauber 1997). Of course, in the absence of microscopy, the distinction between the sickle-shaped cell and other anemias was not conceivable.[*]

Examples abound. What science and technology are able to capture influences what medicine is able to describe. Microbiology, virology, and genetics have all contributed to framing new diagnoses and effacing others. Consumption's transformation into tuberculosis was grounded in microscopy, anchored by the 1882 isolation of the tubercle bacillus by Robert Koch (Daniel 2006);[†] while multiple sclerosis was slowly extirpated from rheumatic disease, constitutional weakness, and paralysis agitans by manual postmortem examination of the brain and spinal cord (Murray 2005).

We don't know what diseases lurk around the corner, what microbe or genetic modification concealed to our eye today will be revealed by technology tomorrow, or similarly, which of the diseases we firmly believe in today will have a completely different form and defining characteristics in a decade or two. The advancement of genetics, proteomics, and molecular profiling progressively exposes new and unexpected diagnoses. What was once breast cancer will now be differentiated, not just on size and grade of the tumor, menopausal status of the patient, nodal involvement or cell type, but also on estrogen or progesterone receptivity and differential gene expression.

Technology has changed our thinking about cancer diagnoses and treatment, with particular gene profiles relating to better or worse prognoses (Sotiriou et al. 2003). Here, Ockham's razor is finely honed, as genomics and proteomics seek to identify the multiplicity of variations present in individual patients, then tailor treatment at the molecular level. Ockham's principle was

---

[*]   The social consequences of this discovery included profound racial prejudices and beliefs about "negro blood" and the necessity of segregation to protect the white race (see Wailoo 1997).

[†]   While Robert Koch, building on the work of René Laennec, provided us with the foundation for the modern definition and conceptualization of tuberculosis, evidence of a tuberculosis-like disease is found in ancient archeological remains in Egypt, in classical Greek texts (when it was known as phthisis), in Hippocratic writings, in the biblical books of Deuteronomy and Leviticus, and in ancient India, China, and the Americas (Daniel 2006).

that groups of things should not be split any more than necessary. But therapeutic necessity seeks very narrow classifications: the greater the specificity of the diagnosis, the more tailored the treatment and the more effective the outcome. Such specificity is clearly enabled by technology.

Yet technology is not independent as it identifies what counts as disease. Technologies are themselves products of their own cultural moment (Wailoo 1997). As Wailoo has described, notably in reference to hematology, disease construction owes much to the technologies of medicine, but not in isolation from medical and cultural context.

The example of chlorosis, a disease that slowly faded from both medical and public repertories at the turn of the twentieth century, provides a useful case in point. Initially presented in social terms, chlorosis was the disease of the delicate woman. It occurred in the overtaxed and the understimulated, the malnourished and the overnourished, the working and the leisure classes. This disease presented in young women as a pallor so extreme as to lend a greenish tinge to the complexion. It was accompanied by tachycardia, shortness of breath, amenorrhea, and gastric difficulties. Wailoo describes three narratives that framed chlorosis and also brought about its demise. The first saw the genesis of the disease in the biological failure of the young woman to adjust to modern society and society's failure to recognize feminine frailty. The concordant treatment resides in careful improvements in physical activity, reduction of external stresses, taking in nourishing food, having frequent bowel movements, and getting ample rest. The second narrative departs from the gender-centered conception to recast chlorosis technologically, according to the hematological profile. The appearance of the chlorotic hemocyte anchored new explanations for the illness. A pale red blood cell visible in the chlorotic patient provided a technological transformation from social to hematological, with "hypochromic anemia" taking the place of chlorosis. Finally, a pharmaceutical approach, born of therapeutic reductionism, anchored chlorosis in the technology of iron metabolism, seeing the green sickness in terms of iron deficiency anemia, and casting a new identity for the nineteenth-century disease. For Wailoo, it is the interaction of technologies with medicine and cultural values that shaped chlorosis's many identities as well as their demise.

Technology is thus not only contained in instrumentation and new forms of imaging or immune assaying; it is also embedded in approaches to knowledge. The science of an era enables some diagnoses and eliminates others. Humoral theory explained disease via the influence of heat, cold, dryness, and moisture on the body. Heat induced relaxation, and cold restriction, of minute fibers of which the body was believed to be constituted (Miller 1962). This could result in diseases such as melancholia. This incapacitating state of sadness, fearfulness, and fatigue of life was attributed to (and etymologically means) "black bile." It was associated with an excess of coldness and dryness (S. Jackson 1978).

Contemporary diagnostic conceptualization bears a similar impact on what can be seen as disease. This "technoscientization," as Clarke and her colleagues have called it, includes the domination of evidence-based medicine in conceptualizing disease. The evidence-based medicine "paradigm" (often now referred to as a "cause" or a "movement") is recent, launched in 1992 by a seminal article published in the *Journal of the American Medical Association*, and written by the Evidence-Based Medicine Working Group, under the chair of Gordon Guyatt. Its recent origins could be traced to Archie Cochrane's 1972 diatribe on effectiveness and efficiency. There, he lamented the absence of measurement of effectiveness of medical interventions and described the randomized controlled trial as a tool for "open[ing] up the new world of evaluation and control" and perhaps saving the National Health Service (Cochrane 1989).

Evidence-based medicine is grounded in a statistical model, which applies formal rules of evidence for evaluating research literature and principles of epidemiology guiding day-to-day clinical practice (Evidence-Based Medicine Working Group 1992). Its central tenet is the hierarchy of evidence, privileging certain kinds of information over others. As postulated by the Evidence-Based Medicine Working Group, "Systematic attempts to record observations in a reproducible and unbiased fashion markedly increase the confidence one can have in knowledge about patient prognosis, the value of diagnostic tests, and the efficacy of treatment. In the absence of systematic observation one must be cautious in the interpretation of information derived from clinical experience and intuition, for it may at times be misleading" (2421).

One important result of the hierarchy of evidence that accompanies evidence-based medicine (EBM) is the way it transforms what counts as disease. Meta-analysis and randomized controlled trials are the highest levels of evidence on the hierarchy and elbow other forms of knowledge out of the way. Things that can be counted and standardized (and therefore evaluated as variables, tested against controls, and statistically synthesized) gain supremacy. Morse has argued that EBM is a politics of ignorance—myopic and exclusionary—that uses Cochrane's standards for evaluating funding for all forms of research. He claims it's a fine sieve that ends up funding drug trials by the powerful and relegating qualitative researchers who are unable to access funds, credibility, and importantly, power (Morse 2006). As Clarke and her colleagues (2003) have pointed out, the information required by EBM (objectified, sanitized, computerized, and statistically analyzed) prevents the clinician from taking the individual body into account. EBM plays an important role in my oft-cited example of overweight's transformation from simple descriptive adjective to disease. Weight is quantitative and imparts implied neutrality (in contrast to the presumed biased subjectivity of self-reported activity or diet) that allows the scales to serve as a proxy measure of wellness, creating a convenient mechanism for understanding corpulence.

Therapeutic technology also frames diagnostic categories. Blaxter (1978) has underlined that the existence of effective treatment refines the understanding of the conditions for which treatment is intended. Wailoo's (1997) discussion of hematological disorders demonstrates the degree to which response to treatment frames diagnostic groups. The administration of liver extracts for pernicious anemia resulted in such a dramatic response that treatment effect determined how patients would be classified. Wailoo calls the treatment a diagnostic tool, "structuring not only medical practice and research, but medical thinking about the identity of the disease" (124). Those cases that did not respond to liver extract were reclassified as "atypical" or "anomalous."

As an extension of this therapy-as-diagnosis, we should reflect back on our discussion of the engines of diagnosis and consider the technological role of pharmaceutical industry interests in the identification of diseases. Returning to female hypoactive sexual desire disorder, we can see how clinical trials of BIMT 17 as an antidepressant had the unexpected result of improved libido in the female participants. This accidental finding is similar to what researchers found when they initially trialed what was to become Viagra. The substance was being tested to determine its efficacy in the reduction of angina, and it was found to lead to a side effect of penile erection in some subjects (Ban 2006). That this discovery coincided with the "discovery" of erectile dysfunction as a debilitating condition affecting over 40 percent of American men is linked closely to the potential market this putative therapeutic agent can satisfy (Lexchin 2006). The success of the trials of flibanserin (BIMT 17) provides a similar technological frame for confirming the presence of FHSDD.

Technology and the Diagnostic Process

Technology tells us things about illness and disease that count for more than what we can say ourselves. In the diagnostic process, technological perspectives are often privileged over the subjective lived experience of the layperson. In the next few paragraphs, I take you on a personal journey to illustrate this point.

On a Thursday, one week in May, I made an appointment to see my general practitioner, Dr. C. When he came to the waiting room to bring me back to his office, we exchanged the regular preexamination banter. "So, how are you doing?" he asked with an appropriate amount of concern in his voice. "Absolutely fantastic! Cured!" I chirruped as we walked into his rooms. He looked at me, mildly confused at this positive response. I had been a regular visitor to his rooms since late January, and the previous week, I was one of his daily call-back patients. I had initially presented with an enigmatic and progressively incapacitating cough. Although I was basically well, the cough was so debilitating that I had been unable to lecture, run, or sleep, all those things that are part of my daily life. I had almost cancelled the overseas trip that was planned for later that month. In the doctor's office, other patients would move to the other side of the waiting room when they heard me hack; I certainly couldn't inflict myself upon airline passengers. I probably would have been too uncomfortable to make the long trip anyway.

My X-ray and blood tests were normal, but a rather banal haemophilus (which may occur as normal flora of the nose and pharynx, but which also may cause illness in the presence of immunosuppression) was initially present in my sputum. I was prescribed antibiotics, with no relenting of the symptoms. A more refined serology test showed exposure (not infection), possibly historical, to pertussis (whooping cough), and a further course of antibiotics was undertaken, with similarly disappointing results. I continued to hack away. Sputum cultures and blood tests were all normal, but I remained ill. Finally, a temporary doctor working the weekend clinic who didn't know me from Adam and probably just wanted me out of his hair, threw diagnostic concern out the window. He prescribed a simple symptomatic treatment of inhaled and oral anti-inflammatory medication, and my cough resolved in a matter of few short hours. There was no diagnosis to label my affliction, but I was better.

Dr. C put his head in his hands as he thought about the trajectory. "I can't believe I didn't try that sooner," he said, embarrassed that I could be "fixed" so easily and yet it had taken almost five months to figure it out. But it was clear to me, and I said this to him, that this specific diagnostic journey was a poignant example of a general trend in medicine, where we subordinate the symptom to the disease and promote the objectivity of science and its associated technological tools to interpret illness.

Leder (1990) laments medicine's current "flight from interpretation" in favor of a form of "immediate apprehension from which hermeneutical subjectivity has been expunged" (20)—in other words, contemporary medicine's reliance on "objective" tests and images such as laboratory values and radiological images. He underlines the rise of technology in the diagnostic process. The appeal of transparent, objective, and irrefutable information about the body—detached from both patient and doctor—intervenes, to a fault, in the diagnostic process.

In addition to overreliance on what Leder has termed the "instrumental," or the purified objectivity of the laboratory finding, a semiotic approach to symptoms further explains the clinical inefficacy of this case. Semiotics is the linguistic study of signs. Simplistically, words (signifiers) represent mental concepts and objects (signifieds). According to Foucault (1963), this semiotic transformation took place in the early nineteenth century with the birth of clinical medicine. Where previously the symptom was the focus of medical practice, now it became a signifier of pathology, the first sign of disease: "Cough, fever, stitch and respiratory difficulties are not pleurisy, which is itself never revealed to the senses . . . but they constitute its essential symptoms" (89). Foucault argues that semiotic theory provides the explanation for clinical observation. The constellation of symptoms points invariably to an underlying disease process. As he explains, "The very heart of illness will give itself up completely in the intelligible syntax of the signifier" (91).

In this context, the symptom is assumed to contain clarity and logic with respect to the disease that necessarily creates it. No longer does the symptom function as an individual phenomenon. Rather, it is linked to interiority and to the disease that is otherwise unseen. The clinician is a detective working to uncover the connection between signifier and disease. In this case study, the pursuit of the hidden condition—autoimmune lung disease or infectious process—was the focus of the interpretive analysis of the abnormal cough. As the doctors delved, they uncovered possible causal agents, but the appropriate treatment resulted in no change in symptoms, belying the relationship between the presumed cause and the clinical complaint. The therapeutic intensity waned with the lack of evidence of disease, even as the cough worsened. The doctors advised me to "wait" or "see how things go" with a reduced sense of immediacy over treatment despite the deterioration in my sense of wellness. I was incapacitated, unable to engage in my normal activities of daily living, and exhausted from unremitting bouts of coughing consuming me by day and waking me and my husband by night.

The fact that my affliction was not a disease was simultaneously a relief and a frustration. On the one hand, it was reassuring that there was no evidence of sarcoidosis, tuberculosis, infection, or malignancy. On the other, because the explanation for my discomfort could not be shown by an objectively visible test result, confirming a known disease, my doctors overlooked symptomatic management. One might argue that these doctors failed in their task, not thinking to provide somatic relief, but I believe they acted coherently within a semiotic disease model, where the symptom is the projection of disease. If the symptom is principally a sign or predictor of an underlying process, it is subordinated to the presumed cause and cannot feature as a clinical entity of its own. Treatment then targets the cause as opposed to the complaint, making the notion of symptomatic treatment incoherent and pushing the doctor toward the irrefutable instrumental (technological) evidence of the disease.

Diagnostic coherence guides clinical interpretation, writes Leder (1990). It is the way the doctor generates provisional diagnoses, tests possible explanations, asks pertinent questions, and prevents each patient encounter from being a start-from-the-beginning random treasure hunt. The more familiar the doctor is with the values and understandings contained in this paradigm, the better will be the potential for effective care. Recognizing the semiotic importance accorded the symptom allows the doctor to diagnose soundly, as well as to identify what to do in the absence of identifiable illness.

Complaints without apparent cause are troublesome. Not only do they fail to signify disease; they frustrate patient and doctor alike. A skeptical clinician may doubt the experiential account of the patient, while a compassionate one may feel impotent and inadequate. The lack of explanation is a threat to medical competence, and suffering can be augmented by anxiety of uncertainty. That the complaint is even real may be doubted, and, in the absence of diagnosis, it may be relegated to the realm of the psychiatric. Indeed, recommendations around medically unexplained symptoms focus on patient emotional management: demonstrating belief in the patient's complaint; giving a positive explanation, including psychological factors; and recommending a return to normal life, as well as cognitive behavioral therapy or antidepressants (Wessely 2002).

My cough provides a useful tool for recognizing the limitation of this approach. One might argue that this cause has a different status than many cases of non-disease-related symptoms, because the clinical complaint is verifiable by the doctor, can be observed and assessed and could be feigned only with difficulty (unlike complaints of "dizziness," "fatigue," or "pain," whose physical presence cannot be witnessed as easily by the clinician). Here the interpretive challenge was not hindered by any disagreement over what had pushed me to see the doctor. What I felt and reported was never denied by the general practitioner or by the specialist, nor did they redefine the narrative as being either nonmedical or nonphysical.

Leder has referred to the "sovereignty of the machine" and the "purified objectivity" conveyed by what he calls "instrumental texts"—which we could perhaps call here, in the context of this chapter, "technological texts." In this case, the sputum and serology reports misled, and the duration of patient suffering was consequently unreasonably prolonged. Here, the doctors sought to treat the disease rather than the patient. The cough was simply a cough. Anti-inflammatory treatment made it go away.

This is what Leder (1990) describes as a pursuit of objective reality and unambiguous results, leading the clinician away from the patient. "The person-as-ill tends to disappear from view when the focus is placed exclusively on certain secondary and tertiary texts. . . . In its attempt to expunge interpretive subjectivity, modern medicine thus threatens to expunge the subject" (20–21).

The reliance on diagnostic imaging, in the United States at least, is fueled by financial imperative. Profit is embedded in procedures, rather than in clinical assessment. A steady increase in the prescription of, and reimbursement for, diagnostic imaging emerges from this principle. With traditional sources of income for doctors being "squeezed," US doctors have been led to seek other revenue streams, among which diagnostic testing features prominently. The cost of radiological imaging is covered by Medicare, rendering the use of X-ray, CT, and MRI attractive to the primary care physician. A kind of medical entrepreneurship has resulted in almost a quarter of MRI machines being owned by non-radiologist physicians, who gain a return on investment by the high volume of the images they generate (Berlin and Berlin 2005).

Screening

There is another side to this story. Up to this point we have considered only the person-as-ill whose illness doesn't find expression in the objective technology of science. But just as salient is the person-as-well whose wellness is refuted by objective findings. David Armstrong's powerful "Rise of Surveillance Medicine" (1995) depicts a medicine concerned with detecting illness before even the individual's health is affected. It is a medicine where symptoms are not coterminous with disease. Rather, disease is considered a silent, unobtrusive potentiality, ready to rear its ugly head in the seemingly healthy when least expected. In surveillance medicine, illness is a complicated set of interrelated states, from apparent healthiness to precursor signs, and finally to overt symptoms of recognized disease.

The idea that ostensibly healthy individuals should subject themselves to medical scrutiny, even in the absence of disease symptoms, dates well back, to at least the mid-nineteenth century. Horace Dobell, in 1861, posited that even well people should have periodic health examinations, because diseases, he believed, were preceded by a state of low health that could provide an opportune window for early treatment. Similarly, George Gould, some years later, suggested that "personal biological examinations" would help doctors both prevent and treat disease before it occurred (Han 1997).

The screening of surveillance medicine extends the diagnostic power to a space *before* disease. The risk factors "are pointers to a potential, yet unformed, eventuality" (Armstrong 1995, 402). As such, both screening and diagnostic events contain a similar transformative power. The abnormal cells, the elevated laboratory values, the unexpected blip on the electrocardiogram—they provide the rationale for treatment or lifestyle modification in those who feel themselves to be well.

Numerous conditions are associated with screening campaigns, some because the result of screening can indeed lead to lifesaving preventative treatment, but there are other reasons as well. Pertinently for this discussion, screening has led to new diagnoses, looking at a set of "pre-" conditions that arguably have their own novel diagnostic status.

One such prediagnosis is prediabetes. This condition is the result of developing tests that are easier to implement and can be used more broadly. A simple blood draw as opposed to a glucose challenge over several hours makes the diagnosis more accessible. Furthermore, a pharmacological treatment, with an eager industry to promote it, also shifts the expectations from what would have previously been a seen as a normal result to create a new disease category with its own set of social consequences (Hunt et al. 2021).

Prediabetes is the name given to people who, when tested for diabetes via the measure of glycated hemoglobin, have an HbA1c measurement between 41 and 49 millimoles per mole, under the usual diagnostic cutoff for type 2 diabetes of 50. A facile but as yet unsubstantiated argument is that being within this range makes a person *at risk* for being diabetic, that being within this range is a "wake-up call." A person can "do something" about their health and avoid diabetes at a later time. This has not been demonstrated; in fact prediabetes, in most cases, does not progress to diabetes (Hunt et al. 2021; Yudkin and Montori 2014). This new diagnostic category, however, has been a gold mine for the pharmaceutical industry, which benefits directly from it, with the prescription of metformin in response to these numbers.

Another social consequence of screening is the identity shift to the patient-in-waiting. Not only is this presumed in the stance toward screening, detailed by Armstrong above; it is also inscribed in the identity of the person thus screened via the idea of *previvorship*. According to Sue Friedman, founder of the Facing Our Risk of Cancer Empowered (FORCE), this term "arose in 2000 from a challenge on the FORCE message board by Jordan, a website regular, who posted, 'I need a label!' . . . As a result, FORCE developed and promoted the term 'cancer previvor' for 'sur*vivor* of a *pre*disposition to cancer.' The term includes people who carry a hereditary mutation, a family history of cancer, or some other predisposing factor who are living with the knowledge of being high-risk." This need for a label, with its accompanying treatment, legitimization, and even possibly stigma, shows how screening, however valorous, brings social as well as clinical impact to the individual.

Surrogate Markers

Prominent in screening tests are surrogate markers, or endpoints. A surrogate marker is a laboratory test result that has a theoretical link with the disease one is trying to detect and prevent. For example, cholesterol, blood pressure, coronary vessel diameter, and left ventricular hypertrophy are among the surrogate markers for heart attacks and heart failure, but none is a true clinical endpoint or evidence of the disease. They are each (and the last two on the list, far more markedly than the earlier examples) linked to diagnosis of the

clinical event (heart disease) and point toward that event, but to different degrees. The marker captures evidence of the process that is thought to underlie
the disease (Temple 1999). High levels of cholesterol can lead to atherosclerosis, which in turn can lead to reduced coronary vessel diameter and ultimately
to myocardial infarction. In principle then, each marker might potentially be
a predictor or indicator of the potential for the clinical outcome one is attempting to prevent. The principle is clear, and the FDA requires that surrogate
markers be "reasonably likely" to predict clinical benefit when they are used
as evidence of clinical utility. In practice, though, surrogate markers are
problematic.

The use of surrogate markers in health screening is a clear nod to the idea
that the human subject is never truly healthy. Further, in clinical research it
is often more useful for marketing than it is valid for patient outcomes (Freemantle and Calvert 2007; Grimes and Schulz 2005). Using surrogate markers
as opposed to clinical endpoints is fraught: medications designed to reduce
cholesterol levels do not necessarily achieve their goal of decreased cardiovascular disease. As one example, in clinical trials, statin drugs (ezetimibe-
simvastatin) lowered serum cholesterol but did not slow the development of
heart disease (atherosclerosis) in patients (Kastelein et al. 2008), their putative purpose.

At a population level, it's easy to see that the risk approach embedded in
surrogate markers has limitations. For example, European cardiovascular guidelines use markers that would classify most adult Norwegians at high risk, despite Norway having one of the world's longest-living and healthiest populations (Getz et al. 2005).

Routine screening seeks to find evidence of disease in a patient who is
presenting for what may be unrelated, and possibly not even clinical, reasons.
Despite the rise in screening as part of health assessment, there is significant
debate about its claimed benefits. Black (2000) has written that detecting sub-
clinical conditions (pseudodiseases) that would have otherwise gone to the
grave with the patient (while not being the cause of death) can result in anxiety, unnecessary treatment, complications, and even actual death. Overdiagnosis, he argues, is a direct result of unnecessary screening, which does not,
in fact, reduce disease-specific mortality. Treating pseudodisease does not im-
prove the odds of those who have real disease. In the case of the Mayo Lung
Project, which tested the effectiveness of intensive screening for lung cancer
against the standard non-screening approach, mortality from lung cancer was

actually *higher* in the screened group than in the control. This is likely because imaging techniques can identify a range of abnormal nodules of unknown clinical significance (Marcus et al. 2006), which are then dealt with aggressively, with all the potential side effects and risk of the treatment.

Screening for disease is practiced with religious fervor, according to Howard Brody (2006), but not always with the acquiescence of the patient. On the surface, it would hardly seem problematic to detect what might be silent for now but disease later. There are many unintended consequences of screening that we should consider, however, including unnecessary medical intervention, living with existential dread, and toxic effects of some treatment. These undesirable effects may extend suffering, rather than alleviate it, not because the person actually lives longer, rather because the prognosis is unaltered by the early diagnosis. There are also occasionally false-positive results to begin with (Jepson 2006).

Political uses of screening are worth noting. We remember a New Zealand election, where an important plank of the incoming government's platform was based on the commonsense notion that because breast cancer screening was an established public health initiative, then prostate cancer screening should be similarly promoted for all men. The vote-generating discourse around this initiative was that men were a neglected underclass who *deserved* screening, despite medical evidence pointing to the fact that screening in asymptomatic men causes harms such as false-positive results, biopsy complications, and overdiagnosis with an unclear impact on cancer mortality (Fenton et al. 2018).

Popular belief is not always easy to shift, with the common belief among the public that screening is "almost always a good idea" even if it does not lead to effective treatment or if the screening reveals pseudodisease. An exaggerated sense of disease risk, the commercial marketing of screening devices and approaches, and inadequate public exploration of how and when screening contributes to well-being are likely at the root of these beliefs (Schwartz et al. 2004).

Other markers serve a quite different purpose and instead of stigmatizing, legitimize illness experiences. A particular case in point is the genetic markers observed in veterans of nuclear testing. One cohort of nuclear test veterans, in 1957, observed as many as nine nuclear detonations in the mid–Pacific Ocean (Kiribati, Malden Island, and Christmas Island). A number of the veterans who witnessed these detonations have reported a range of medically unexplained symptoms: genetic disorders among their descendants and increased incidence of multiple myeloma, gastric and respiratory disorders, and arthritis. The claims made by these veterans have been difficult to prove, as much of the documentary evidence of their exposure is controlled by the parties the veterans claim are culpable: the British and NZ navies (Trundle 2010).

Genetic testing of 50 individuals from within this group, as compared to 50 matched controls has demonstrated chromosomal damage (Wahab et al. 2008). Translocation and extraordinarily complex chromosomal rearrangements such as those viewed in these tests are generally suggestive of radiation exposure. These biological markers (chromosome translocation frequency) became an important evidentiary tool for those servicepeople seeking compensation for themselves and their families on the basis of radiation exposure during the tests. Here, the genetic marker is not a stigma, as in the previous examples; rather, it is a tangible indication of liability, according to these veterans. It legitimizes their suffering and their anxieties and opens the way for compensation.

Other markers may be used in occupational health to identify early effects of toxic agents in the body (exposure) or individual predispositions to be more or less harmed by chemical exposure (susceptibility). Although such monitoring is part of many occupational health and safety strategies, it raises ethical concerns about workers' well-being, including job loss, stigmatization, reassignment, and insurance/mortgage ineligibility (Caux et al. 2007).

Genetic Discrimination

Disease potential is a salient means of social control and is amplified by the ever-expanding technical access to new screening tools. Lippman (1991) has described how genetic risk, in particular, captures an increasingly wide array of social concerns:

> Using the metaphor of blueprints, with genes and DNA fragments presented as a set of instructions, the dominant discourse describing the human condition is reductionist, emphasizing genetic determination. It promotes scientific control of the body, individualizes health problems and situates individuals increasingly according to their genes. Through this discourse, which is beginning seriously to threaten other narratives, clinical and research geneticists and their colleagues are conditioning how we view, name and propose to manage a whole host of disorders and disabilities. Though it is only one conceptual model, "genetics" is in-

creasingly identified as *the* way to reveal and explain health and disease, normality and abnormality. (18)

Genetic screening becomes a modern/counter-modern form of biological determinism, which describes the supposed social risk presented by this or that particular profile, giving individuals the potential to respond to their future and make reproductive decisions. Nevertheless, the genetic movement has difficulty moving past its eugenic roots.

The potential to detect genetic predispositions for disease, for example, may lead to many discriminatory practices reminiscent of eugenic "selective breeding" and "racial hygiene." This is notable in insurance coverage, where genetic testing, as well as (one presumes) technologies yet to come, provides a new range of risk profiles that insurers are loath to assume, incorporating premodern notions of fatalism (Kerr and Cunningham-Burley 2000).

Prenatal diagnosis is another area where technology is playing an increasingly wide role. From amniocentesis to chorionic villus sampling and nuchal translucency, tests reveal the genotype and potential abnormalities. Regardless of the discourse surrounding testing, be it reassurance that the baby is going to be normal or control over what types of babies can be born, the pragmatic outcome of prenatal diagnosis is generally geared toward selective abortion and the elimination of fetuses with genetic defects (Lippman 1991). I am not here expressing a judgment about selective abortion, rather underlining the fact that the outcome of diagnostic technology, in this case, emphasizes medical rather than social diagnosis and intervention. This raises the question, for example, is Down syndrome (one prevalent prenatal diagnostic object) an undesirable condition or simply a variant of the range of ways of being? The stigmatization of the individual with Down syndrome focuses on perceived negative potentials (present in all unborn, unraised children, whose intellectual capacities are neither known nor fixed) rather than on other aspects of individual personality.

Privileging certain traits via technologies of prenatal selection presents a new eugenics, putatively based on neoliberal, individual choice rather than governmental coercion or force. It has been suggested, however, that there is an implicit coercion emerging from medical authority and discriminatory beliefs about disability (Raz 2009). Being a carrier of a genetic marker for a particular diagnosis may result in discriminatory practices. Screening programs, such as the Dor Yeshorim premarital genetic testing for potential spouses in ultra-

Orthodox Jewish communities, results in the reinforcement of stigma of those who are presumed to be genetic carriers (Raz and Vizner 2009).

Kerr and Cunningham-Burley (2000) maintain that genetic testing reflects modernist claims about knowledge and control. The technologies may yet be superficial and uncertain, but they are approached, for a variety of reasons, with a certainty and an imperative toward action. "Risk estimates become definitive diagnoses which form part of a chain of diagnostic procedures, starting with counseling and proceeding to abortion, prophylactic treatment or further monitoring" (289).

Hope

Technology cannot be viewed simply as a tool of social control, ensuring patient compliance and reinforcing the hegemonic "medical-industrial complex with dark motives and dependent victims" (Timmermans and Berg 2003, 98) playing a game of biological or genetic selection. Technology is not constructed in a vacuum; it is infiltrated and shaped by medical beliefs, professional priorities, lay and social anxieties. In addition to classifying, discriminating, and screening, technology also clearly buttresses therapeutic directions.

Timmermans and Berg (2003) posit that sociology has much to offer technology when disciplinary boundaries are put to one side and insights about autonomy, patienthood, and embodied experience can be presented to technology designers. While I have discussed the potential for technology to trump embodied experience, and for technological findings to dominate the clinical hermeneutic, we can equally invest great hope in the potential that technology may offer.

Tragically, Suzanne Fleischman (1999), whose reflections on the language of disease I have cited regularly throughout this book, died a young woman. Her essay—part personal documentary, part exercise in medical semantics, as she described it—drew upon her experience of a rare (and ultimately fatal) illness. In it, technology was paradoxically both the signatory to her death warrant and vector of hope: "My dreams would conjure up kaleidoscopic images of chromosomes, gene products, transcription factors, and Freudian fragments of damaged DNA longing for repair. Perhaps one of those dreams will engineer a technology for fixing chromosomal breaks in hematopoietic stem cells" (5).

The technology of diagnosis has many potentials. It can emancipate and oppress, clarify and obfuscate, or legitimize medical attitudes and identities (Wailoo 1997, 45). For Fleischman, and indeed for anyone who has endured the transformative insult of the malignant diagnosis, technology is an important life raft. Each test and each therapeutic undertaking raises hope in the remote possibility that an explanation (or even better, a solution) will issue from the next new finding. This may, in part, explain the American fascination described by Schwartz and colleagues (2004) with technological profiles, however imprecise. They are like the pill I imagined as a little girl, the one that science would certainly discover for me, that would let me live forever. Science is always ever just on the brink of solving our problems, I believed, among which mortality is probably the highest priority.

Hope also emerges in the technologies of chronic illness, where instrumental understandings of the body contribute to self-awareness and identity. For example, women who had bone scans to detect osteoporosis wanted these images, whatever stories they told. They believed the images revealed an inner truth about themselves that was not otherwise accessible. This fostered new understandings about themselves and their body image. In this case, the bone scan provided a view of the body-object in ways that reorganized their body space and gave different meanings to their experiences of embodiment (Reventlow, Hvas, and Malterud 2006).

Genetic technology enables women with BRCA1/2 mutations to identify their marked increased risk of breast and ovarian cancer. Women with these mutations can choose to have both breasts removed even in the absence of any sign of disease. One cohort study over six years showed a reduction in breast cancer of 95 percent in those who elected for double mastectomy (Rebbeck et al. 2004). Opting for mastectomy is nonetheless a difficult choice. Not all women who are BRCA1/2 positive will have cancer, although the risk is high.

An important theme in syndromes such as the medically unexplained symptom and chronic fatigue is the hope that technology will transform suffering into a legitimized medical condition rather than an elusive and invisible state of maladaptation. When the laboratory test or the radiographic image concords with the phenomenological experience of illness, the individual has access to a biomedical explanation that in turn provides social recognition of their suffering (Hydén and Sachs 1998). One important function served by diagnostic testing is visual revelation; that which is neither visually inscribed on the body (it doesn't "show") nor previously validated by medicine gains substance via its inscription in visual imaging. The CT provides, as one informant explained, "solid proof. It [isn't] just aches and pains anymore" (Rhodes et al. 1999, 1194). What the patient had "been saying to her doctor could not be heard until, to her joy, it could be seen" (1195). This position of hope reverberates with the case I presented of my own cough. Being able to "see" the illness in its scientized existence would have made my condition real and treatable, as opposed to the unfortunate dilemma it became within an objectified, diagnostically organized medicine.

Hope is fueled not only by technology's potential to cure but also by its status as a commodity in the free market. Consumer longing for eternal good health and belief in science as an objective yet beneficent purveyor of worthwhile technologies is a practical marketing object in commodity culture. Archie Alexander (2007) describes the United States as the "land of medical imaging opportunity, where anyone can participate in the ultrasound imaging experience" (1). Technological systems can be purchased, and technological experiences can be marketed outside of medical prescription. The ultrasound about which Alexander writes goes beyond its usual diagnostic use to become the plaything of the rich consumer. Tom Cruise, we understand, purchased his own ultrasound machine in order to "visit" his gestating son whenever the mood struck him.

I have elsewhere described how the previously acquiescent patient has received access to information formerly restricted to medicine as a result of new media. This e-scaping is complemented by the increasing presence of diagnostic technologies as consumer products available outside of medical networks. Fetal "keepsake" imaging," for example, is a commercial appropriation of the diagnostic imaging to offer expectant parents a prenatal view of their infant. Companies like Hello Baby provide elective, nonmedical access to an ultrasound view of their baby. The FDA has strongly discouraged the use of ultrasound for nonmedical purposes, and commercial providers may violate the law if it is not medically prescribed (American Pregnancy Association 2023).

The place of technology in medicine is immense, and the glimpse contained in these few thousand words barely scratches the surface of its impact in diagnosis. I have not, for example, explored the role of technology in lay and professional education and communication. Nor have I discussed the fuzzy line between genetic enhancement and genetic manipulation that technology offers. What once might have been considered a disadvantage (a "Jewish nose," for example) might, in the presence of the ability to "fix" it, become a disease or a condition worthy of repair, perhaps on the basis that it creates an inferiority complex (see Gilman 1991). I have not even touched upon the economics of diagnostic technology that feature in the design and use of diagnostic tests and the treatments that ensue (Laking, Lord, and Fischer 2006).

Technology is not freely allocated and produces dramatic differences in ethnic, demographic, and national diagnostic trends. What we are capable of diagnosing depends not only on our technological ability to diagnose but also on the availability of the equipment to access the technology. In developing countries, in remote and rural areas, and in underprivileged neighborhoods, what we take for granted as tools for diagnostic confirmation remain inaccessible. Even simple biomechanical injuries might never be named in nations such as the Cook Islands or Tokelau, where the X-ray is the only imaging technology available. A CT or an MRI might be as far as three days away by slow boat.

The story of technology's contribution to diagnosis within a social and cultural frame does not end with this chapter. It is a story yet to be told, given the ever-changing technologies available for diagnostic purposes. It is, however, a story that can be generically recognized as we study the sociology of diagnosis, because it is an important framing device in diagnostic categories and concordant therapeutic reactions.

CHAPTER SEVEN

COVID-19 as a Sociological Phenomenon

The virus implicated in a mysterious outbreak of pneumonia in central China is in a class of pathogens that are a growing player in global infectious disease epidemics.

The *Wall Street Journal* reported this week that Chinese scientists identified a new type of so-called coronavirus as a possible cause of the outbreak in the city of Wuhan, where 59 people have been sickened, with seven in critical condition.

Chinese authorities say they have found coronavirus in patients, but haven't confirmed it as the underlying cause of the illnesses. But virologists and epidemic experts say it is likely.   MCKAY (2020)

Since the first edition of this book, in 2011, diagnosis has become more real in many ways. Not only has it continued to occupy an ever-growing space in the popular imagination, as a universal form of explanation, a narrative trope, and a source of entertainment, but we've also come to understand its importance in public health: how particular diagnoses (COVID-19) compel particular actions. Even in a popular era of diagnosis, only a few years ago, the contemporary familiarity with R values, viral variants, and PCR assays would have been surprising.

At the same time, diagnosis has also become more real as a sociological topic, with a deeper exploration of diagnosis as a social and cultural phenomenon. These two positions might seem oppositional or at least paradoxical. As the materiality of viral infection infringes on our day-to-day lives in sometimes catastrophic ways, how does sociology (the sociology of diagnosis) offer a helpful and meaningful way of understanding disease? In this penultimate chapter, I use COVID-19 as a diagnosis of interest. I show how it too can be beneficially understood by the "explanatory repertoire of sociology" (Weinberg 2020, 2) and how precisely, it is shaped by the same social forces as any other diagnosis.

COVID-19, at first glance, might seem to be more "real" than many other diagnoses. COVID-19 is a "thing," "we understand it," one might argue. We know its causative agent, its symptoms, its consequences. We see pictures of it in the media with its striking, blossom-like, and usually red-stained ultrastructural morphology. Notwithstanding—and even with the extreme material consequences that COVID-19 has had on individuals and on entire populations—it too has porous and non-ontological boundaries. It has a distinct social existence, which the scholar should subject to critical analysis along with its clinical and public health challenges. It is a lesson in the sociology of diagnosis par excellence.

But like any other diagnosis, before COVID-19 could become what it is, it had to be "seen." Now this reference to seeing is not simply to microscopy but to its recognition as something that should be subjected to microscopy. I refer back to the example I have used throughout this book: if the disease had first manifested in a rural, underserved community and no transmission took place outside of one isolated farm family, say, the absence of a significant "cluster" (an epidemiological term to which all have become familiar in the past years) might make the pursuit of genetic sequencing an unthought-of task. The virus could exist in nature but remain unrecognized and without diagnosis. The existence of diagnosis, thus, is completely dependent upon a context in which the condition appears and the degree to which it raises concern.

I've described a compelling example of the cluster as sociocultural phenomenon in relation to the "discovery" of Lyme disease (see chapter 1). Numerous other diseases (PTSD, HIV, fibromyalgia, Alzheimer disease, and so on) similarly owe their recognition to social health movements and individual efforts (see, for example, Brown et al. 2004; Callard and Perego 2021; Chaufan et al. 2012; P. Conrad 2005; W. Scott 1990).

With this in mind, we might consider simply how pandemics "made" diagnosis a system for medicine. The *International Classification of Diseases (ICD)* was developed in a different era precisely to track cross-border contagion of infectious disease, which hadn't been quite so imperative in previous eras. As transportation became more effective between nations, the spread of diseases also increased. Given that sick people could now survive the duration of travel between countries, these travelers served as vectors to transport disease from one nation to another. To monitor the health of nation-states and the progression of disease, there needed to be a consistent means for referring to communicable diseases (Bowker 1996). Without recognizing illnesses in the same way across national boundaries, a pandemic is not possible. A stable diagnostic classification system is thus at the heart of the COVID-19 pandemic (Jutel 2021).

Just how stable can a viral diagnosis be? Influenza is a good example of how fluid a seemingly bounded diagnosis can be; it provides a model for understanding the similar elusive fluidity of the COVID-19 diagnosis (see Jutel 2013). A virus changes forms, vectors, and names. Spanish flu, swine flu, bird flu: Are they all influenza? They are if we define influenza in relation to their membership of the family Orthomyxoviridae, "the genome of which consists of segmented negative-sense single-strand RNA segments" (Arbeitskreis Blut 2009). This technical description of the genome is always accompanied by an explanation of the rapid evolution and variability of influenza strains. What makes it one class of disease is actually the fact that it is so variable. The diagnosis is based on similarity and on difference—or more precisely, on differentiability.

COVID-19 too has myriad variant forms. With each new variant (be it the B.1.1.7 "UK variant" and all its mutations, the B.1.351, Delta, Omicron, or any of the dozens of others),* tiny alterations in the sequence of nucleic acid have taken place over time, as the virus meets new hosts and spreads in new contexts, increasing how tightly it might bind to its receptor and enter human cells (Lee 2021).

When we consider that the so-called UK variant has 23 mutations (Lee 2021) from the original Wuhan strain, we might ask whether it is still the same virus or is now a different disease. The sociologist of diagnosis would probably ask what social function is served by differentiating one strain from the other. Even between writing my first draft of this chapter and the final version, new strains both come into being and become "visible." As I write today, we are tussling with the Omicron strain and wondering what Sigma or Theta will resemble.

Should a diagnosis be made based on the relationship of the virus to Wuhan or on the basis of potential treatment or impact? That a particular vaccination works or doesn't work is part of the social work of diagnosis. This leads, perhaps, to what Blaxter proposed, a kind of social taxonomy of prescriptive diagnosis; the disease must be identified for the treatment to be prescribed: the Pfizer-preventable COVID-19, the AstraZeneca one, the Johnson & Johnson

---

* And given the speed of mutation, who knows what we'll be talking about by the time this book goes to press! The reader can use this paragraph as a form of historical evidence as to the day on which I wrote these lines.

one. Diagnostic labels are shaped according to what social action we are primed, or able, to take. Response to treatment can determine diagnosis.

By labeling a condition as same or as different, we have means for variously controlling community spread or inciting action. That health officials have chosen not to create different diagnostic labels in this case reflects the importance of population compliance with public health initiatives. To see the variants as different would complicate control. But at the same time, the variants also impose particular forms of social and political control. The appearance of Delta in Australia led to severe lockdowns even in the presence of only a few cases, a different situation than the presence of earlier strains. New Zealand went into total lockdown after the identification of three Delta community cases.

If we turn to the diagnostic process, as our model compels us to, access to diagnosis depends sometimes on a diagnostic test and other times, on a case definition. In a non-pandemic year, for example, an influenza diagnosis would most likely come from case definition: Does the patient have the requisite aches, pains, fever, and exposure? From a surveillance perspective, the case definition is made up of the criteria used to count cases consistently and ultimately to monitor public health. It is rare for an individual to be tested for influenza in the outpatient setting and usually isn't clinically necessary. But as all readers of this chapter will know, testing for COVID-19 became a public health imperative for counting cases. On the particular day that I am writing, New Zealand is priding itself on a low-case day. It is not just epidemiologists who muse about whether there has been a drop in actual testing numbers to explain these low case numbers. People on the street know to ask such questions. In any case, regardless of whether we are talking about diagnosis via case definition or lab test, its social contingency is constant.

The case definition is "a set of standard criteria for classifying whether a person has a particular disease, syndrome, or other health condition. . . . Use of an agreed-upon standard case definition ensures that every case is equivalent, regardless of when or where it occurred, or who identified it" (CDC 2012, 1–20). Counting cases is the job of the epidemiologist, and cases are identified by meeting particular criteria. The step is not always taken from criteria to confirmatory laboratory tests, however.

In the case of COVID-19, depending on country, swabs and PCR were more likely to be implemented than in the case of common influenza, but one point is clear: case definition may or may not capture the reality of the infection. As many as 40 percent of COVID-19 cases are asymptomatic (Oran and Topol 2020).

But back to the case definition. Looking at the CDC definition above, the generic descriptions of symptoms used in a case definition is "agreed upon" and so immediately confirms its social nature. The word "agreement" signifies that either a consensus was derived or there was some other manner of alignment among human actors (Aronowitz 2001).

But from country to country, COVID-19 case definitions are not uniform. Case definitions shift over time (as I discuss in greater depth below), but I make my argument on the basis of the case definitions in place in 2021, at the time I wrote these words. They have undoubtedly changed since, which should further confirm the elusive and consensus-based nature of diagnosis.

The World Health Organization's case definition at the time of writing focuses on acute onset of fever and cough or "acute onset of any three or more of the following signs or symptoms: fever, cough, general weakness/fatigue, headache, myalgia, sore throat, coryza, dyspnoea, anorexia/nausea/vomiting, diarrhoea, altered mental status" (2020).

But a glance at my home country's definition doesn't make mention of fever: "Any acute respiratory infection with at least one of the following symptoms: new or worsening cough, sore throat, shortness of breath, coryza—head cold (eg, runny nose, sneezing, post-nasal drip), anosmia—loss of sense of smell" (Oran and Topol 2020).

Both case definitions are followed by red flags that should increase suspicion. In New Zealand, this would be some sort of connection to the national border; for the WHO, residing, working, or traveling in or to a high-risk area.

Even within a single organization or nation, the case definition will morph over time, as I said above. Again, to return to New Zealand, in May 2020, the case definition *did* include the fever that no longer features in its definition: at this earlier stage, a fever ($\geq 38°C$) "AND/OR any acute respiratory infection with at least one of the following symptoms: cough, sore throat or shortness of breath" (Ministry of Health 2020). So, even case definitions are fluid, shifting to catch up with a rapidly mutating virus and reflecting changing human understandings of the disease.

Regardless of the material reality of the virus, whether one will be diagnosed with any disease depends on standards and social agreement. This extends beyond case definitions to diagnostic testing. Tests are seen to be more objective than a clinical diagnosis, but they are not infallible. They may be sensitive but not specific, specific but not sensitive: the "false" positives and negatives.

In the early days of the COVID-19 pandemic, testing was mainly on hospitalized patients. The more testing rates increased, the more the pretest probability (or likelihood that the person tested would be infected) decreased.

While one could retort that a novel diagnosis is bound to change, that its fluid identity is the result of our developing understanding rather than an example of how diagnosis works as social agreement, any one of a number of other disease examples could be used in its stead. Indeed, we develop new understandings of most conditions over time—understandings that will shift again, in due course. They can be anything from the still poorly understood chronic fatigues and chronic pains to much the more mundane category of obesity.

As I discussed in chapter 2, the diagnosis of obesity was, in the nineteenth century, based on qualitative assessment instead of measurement. A clinician would note "excess adiposity" (Jutel 2006), and scales were rarely involved. They were expensive and not necessarily part of a doctor's armory. Indeed, as height and weight charts started to make their appearance, triggered by their use in an actuarial setting, doctors resisted their incorporation in the clinical assessment. By the 1980s, body mass index became the gold standard of assessment, despite the fact that it was a population measure and not a measure of adiposity, an example of the well-known "ecological fallacy."*

But Kuczmarski and Flegal (2000) have shown in their historical analysis of criteria for the definition of the ideal weight, standards have varied no fewer than 18 times between 1942 and 2000. Obesity is a moving target, not necessarily based on deeper understanding or on the forward progress of science. Numerous factors, many of which are not clinical, reshape our criteria each time we turn our eyes to a diagnostic category.

Changing definitions of disease are also grounded in contest and challenge the boundaries of medical authority, reflecting how diagnosis is a coveted social object that shapes the landscape of illness, confirms a hierarchy of authority (a powerful disease namer and a submissive "patient"), and authorizes the distribution of services and allowances.

Whether the diagnosis opens doors via the resources it provides or closes them as a result of the stigma it confers, it will shape the experience of illness.

---

* Ecological fallacies are "untested inferences about individual-level relationships from aggregate data" (Firebaugh 2015, 865).

The hierarchy of diseases that Album and his colleagues have written about (Album et al. 2017; Album and Westin 2008) links perceived "disease prestige" by medical professionals to diagnoses where medical heroism can play a role, where technologically sophisticated and invasive therapeutics can wrest a young person from the jaws of death or disability. In contrast, diseases that are chronic, nonspecific, and have less visible treatments (or older patients) are less worthy. Myocardial infarction and brain tumors are at the top of the hierarchy, with fibromyalgia and anxiety at the bottom.

A stigma may be associated with particular diagnoses. It may be overt, based on a belief in the social unacceptability of any one of a number of low-prestige disorders: fibromyalgia (a disease you have to "fight" to get [Dumit 2006]), epilepsy (Scambler 2009), HIV (Mahajan et al. 2008), mental illness (Dinos et al. 2004), obesity (Puhl and Brownell 2003), and so on. The stigma may be overt, and from external sources, or "felt," leading to concealment by the individual thus diagnosed (Scambler 2009).

Some diagnoses have different valence at different times. In normal times, to have influenza is neither a blight on one's identity nor a generally accepted reason for quarantine. The "flu" is a familiar trope. We call it by a nickname ("flu" being a shortened form of the formal diagnosis "influenza"), and we often mention it in jest, minimizing a colleague's complaint as merely "man flu." However, when the words "epidemic" and "pandemic" surface, usually uttered by health authorities, this benign seasonal visitor becomes something quite different.

Bird flu (H5N1) and swine flu (H1N1), for example, are different from seasonal influenza. These are both influenza A viruses. They are categorized by specific proteins on the surface of the virus: the hemagglutinin (H) and neuraminidase (N) of which there are numerous subtypes that can be arranged in different configurations (CDC 2009b). Even though influenza mutates every season, these two strains are seen to merit special recognition (and indeed, discrete diagnostic status) because they've jumped vectors (from an animal to a human) and because of their potential severity. The World Health Organization reports the mortality rate from person-to-person bird flu infection may be upwards of 60 percent (n.d.).

When a bird flu epidemic emerged in 2004, anxiety spread quickly. Even in the absence of obvious human-to-human transmission (CDC 2008), the idea of an invasive "other" rapidly took hold in media representations of the virus. Western media depicted peasant farmers living among their fowl and slaughtering chickens in their backyards (Stephenson and Jamieson 2009), and the emphasis was on how different the context was from that of the "civilized" Westerner. This mirrored the fear of "Asian invasion," further mixing the idea of immigration with the idea of contagion (Nerlich and Halliday 2007). Descriptions of the avian flu used invasion metaphors, usually military: "Like enemy troops moving into place for an attack, the bird flu known as A(H5N1) has been steadily advancing," and "diseases don't stop at state lines, any more than they do at national borders" (in Hanne and Hawken 2007, 95).

In a similar vein, anti-immigration lobbyists responded to the 2009 H1N1 (swine flu) epidemic by latching on to a presumed Mexican origin of the disease to fuel their campaigns (see, for example, Judicial Watch 2009; Wooldridge 2009). In popular imagination, the H1N1 pandemic of 2009 started in a Mexican hacienda where pigs, dogs, humans, and other mammals mingled in a primitive manner. But cases of a swine-origin influenza A were simultaneously described in Mexico and in Southern California in early April (CDC 2009b). It was just as likely that the epidemic started in an American split-level.

The meanings given to influenza in pandemic times are thus different from those of the influenza of early winter. State and national borders take on meaning that they didn't previously. To be ill is to either be an invader or a tainted citizen. Being acknowledged as a "case" may blemish the individual thus diagnosed. To be an early case at the heart of a cluster or to return from Europe or the United States with the virus was to release one's claim to be a citizen, a team player (Jutel 2021). During COVID-19 times, health officials also turn their attention to their citizenry, worried that the condemnation of infected individuals will force sick people underground, a far greater risk to the wider population than to be diagnosed.

In New Zealand, a flurry of social media responses to the first community cluster after a previously successful elimination campaign was so divisive as to generate a call from the minister of health at his daily press briefing to stop spreading rumors: "Not only was it harmful and dangerous, it was totally and utterly wrong" (Coughlan 2020). This phenomenon was observed more widely, with "a 'witch hunt' hysteria" fueling discrimination and hate directed toward infected individuals but also, as many readers may remember, an anti-Chinese discrimination going as far as to target Chinese restaurants in countries very far from any pandemic epicenter (Sotgiu and Dobler 2020).

I've mentioned above a range of stigmatized diagnoses; it's important to recognize that any diagnosis creates a social reaction, with varying degrees of association with character traits: gout may be seen as a sign of gluttony and sloth, lung cancer of addiction and poor self-control, and so on. Historically, the association of tuberculosis with the dreamy creative and of chlorosis with elite-class femininity are examples, seems quaint to our twenty-first-century sensibility but not unlike the associations of our era, which will be similarly quaint to readers a century or two from now. History simply provides a critical distance that allows us to recognize the values contained in what we take for granted as "truth" in any given era.

Interestingly as well, COVID-19 not only stigmatized; it was a powerful unifier. Appeals to solidarity were a rallying cry during the pandemic. From the "Team of five million effort" (Cheng 2020) and "We're all in this together" (*Stuff* 2020) to "Unite against COVID-19" (New Zealand Government 2020), "Stay connected" (Government of Ireland 2020), and "Join the effort" (Government of Canada 2020), the slogans of public health and of politics concentrated on the collective and on the nation.

Paradoxically, the isolation imposed by COVID-19, into a "bubble" in New Zealand, a "household group" in Scotland, or the "rule of 6" in England, introduced citizens into a new network, one that explores connections and contacts, casual and close. As soon as a case was identified, a close analysis of where the person had been, who they passed in the corridor, who they embraced, and or with whom they shared a meal is triggered. The people thus revealed assume a shared identity, and in solidarity (albeit, usually imposed), they too go into isolation, have a test, become part of the network. So, it's a situation of being simultaneously together and apart. During COVID times, illness is no longer a solitary burden to shoulder; it's a sign to join the ranks and head to the local testing center. COVID-19 is a national challenge, one that binds individuals to the spirit of the nation.

Nations are never natural divisions. Like diagnoses, they are a form of social categorization, where historical, cultural, traditional, political, and other forces break the natural continuum into chunks that can be understood, defended, and serve some sort of purpose. Nation-states are created, for the most part, not along natural boundaries, languages, or ethnicities but rather by subtle gestures that enable us "to understand the assumptions of the daily news" (15). As Billig describes in his *Banal Nationalism* (1995), little things create the nation: the use of words like "here" and "us" and "them." These words focus the attention on the imaginary thing that "we" are and that allows "the media of mass communication [to bring] the flag across the contemporary hearth." This "national first-person plural" serves as a continuous reminder of the nation-state, no matter which one we/you/they belong to. Diagnosis serves as one of the "daily, unmindful reminders of the nationhood in the contemporary, established nation-state" (174).

Be it influenza, SARS, HIV, or today, COVID-19, these diagnoses punctuate nationhood by the fact that their causative agents disrespect the "invented permanency" (Billig 1995, 29) of the nation. Their incursions compel the state to respond, to define itself as distinct and unified. While reminders such as the first-person plural may be banal in non-pandemic times, they become not-so-banal in times of viral threat. It is a unification borne of crisis and couched as such in metaphor and in description. While the banal "we" and "us" persists, so too does the accrual of metaphors of unification. The external threat of disease becomes affixed to other nation-states. A favorite military metaphor of UK ministers used during the current COVID-19 pandemic is of the population "being all in it together," which hearkens to the repeated popular representation of World War II as shared experience of the civilian and the military, as in the quintessential example, *In Which We Serve*, directed by Noel Coward (Lacey, Jutel, and Kelly 2020).

I promised a return to the idea of diagnostic contest. Firmly linked to the consequences of diagnosis, the welcome ones as well as the stigmatizing ones, there can be a tussle around diagnostic labels that has an ongoing effect on what labels are accepted and which are discarded, and which are integrated into official diagnostic structures. Disease recognition, as Phil Brown has called it, is the way in which particular ailments are considered worthy of diagnostic status. It is a fraught and alienating process when the control over recognition is held in one location to which not all have access.

COVID-19 too is open to such contest. It's not that people are claiming COVID-19 in the absence of viral confirmation; it's that patient experience of it does not always match medical descriptions of its outcomes. "Long COVID," or "long-haul COVID," has been identified by numerous people recovering from a COVID-19 infection but was viewed with some skepticism by the medical community. Pivotal here is the illness-disease dichotomy. The medical description of COVID-19 and its consequences is at odds with the patient experience. As I mentioned in chapter 4, Callard and Perego (2021) have explained that recognition of long COVID, or the persistence of COVID-19 symptoms beyond the acute infectious period, was driven by advocacy from people suffering from ongoing symptoms weeks after their initial infection. The question of how such an ailment would be considered diagnostically—is it COVID-19 related or an expression of a more generic post-viral fatigue syndrome?—remains at the moment of writing, unresolved.

Callard and Perego argue that this may be the first totally patient-constructed diagnosis, developed with the networks of social media, and they believe that it may shift assumptions about diagnostic discovery. I would counter that while social media is a new mechanism, there are two flaws in this argument. The first is that although the individuals suffering from what they call long COVID are indeed pivotal in bringing awareness to the condition, they will ultimately be out in the cold when it comes to its confirmation as a diagnosis. Confirmation of diagnostic status remains in the hands of the institutions. When "long COVID," or some other configuration of this name, becomes part of the *ICD* or an extension of a classification or coding document available for use by diagnosticians, then it will be a diagnosis. For the moment, it is an example of a lay-driven disease awareness phenomenon, not of a diagnostic creation.

But second, I counter by saying that this is not the first time. We saw it in the case of Lyme disease (Aronowitz 1991). And in Taiwan, the described condition "autonomic imbalance" (Chen 2021) is another lay-driven condition that has been offered clinical meaning in Western and traditional medicine settings, albeit not yet with full diagnostic status. But neither of these examples undermine the importance of these observations about long COVID.

Long COVID holds a particular place in the hierarchy of fatigue. It is not psychosomatic, and it is certainly not chronic fatigue or fibromyalgia, argue its sufferers. There is pushback against the idea that it is *not* CFS, a diagnosis somehow less valorous. I have already explained that unexplained symptoms are often perceived as not "real." Long COVID sufferers are eager to ensure that they are not seen in that light.

We can return to Phil Brown's 1995 "Naming and Framing" (1995), where he underlined the importance of laypeople, often central to the discovery of diseases and conditions. Such lay-initiated discoveries are only conflictual in the degree to which they are part only of the illness experience or part of a shared experience of the condition.

Conclusion

COVID-19 provides us with an exercise in sociology. It shows us how the seemingly neutral disease label is a rich social phenomenon, dependent upon consensus and power, linked to resources and therapeutics, stigmatizing and valorous, and a trigger for myriad social actions. We can see how diagnostic processes are similarly social, even in the presence of the pretty pomander of COVID-19.

Any named condition has a social existence, and social consequences, alongside the physical or psychological disorder. The critical diagnosis scholar can find that social content. In the conclusion, I propose a social model of diagnosis (revised) to aid in assembling social reflection about diagnosis.

Diagnosis is a resource for medical sociology as well as a topic (Weinberg 2020). As we explore diagnoses via the social model, we see clearly many of the topics of importance to the medical sociologist: the location of power, the distribution of resources, the line between "badness and sickness" (Conrad and Schneider 1980), lay discovery, contest, and so on. Because diagnosis is a social agreement, entailing social consequences, its study can provide important insights into the social context in which such agreements are entered or in which such consequences occur. Diagnosis captures medicine, in a kind of freeze-frame, showing us what matters in the exercise of medicine and the experience of health and disease.

Directions for the Sociology of Diagnosis

> People who suffer from compassion fatigue often have high and unrealistic ideas about how they can help others. They believe they should be able to give endlessly, heal everyone and always be right. . . . This can also lead to frustration or anger in workplaces such as hospitals or rest homes where there is a high level of fatigue or stress. . . . [C]ertain personalities are also more vulnerable to compassion fatigue.　　　VENITIA SHERSON (2010)

The term "compassion fatigue" was first mooted in a Spanish nursing journal: "Contact with disease and death, with the suffering of the others . . . demands great psychological stability and creates tremendous stress in those professionals that live day to day with their patients" (*Revista de enfermeria* 1989, 9), the journal's editor wrote, pleading with nurses to seek help and support. Following in its wake, publications in the fields of medicine and other caring professions started speaking about compassion fatigue. They focused on the exhaustion and psychological distress that resulted from the burden of caring for others who suffer (Booth 1991; Cassidy 1991; Joinson 1992). This burnout, or psychological exhaustion, was cast as a disorder. Joinson (1992) described its symptoms to nurses: "You forget or lose things or have a shorter attention span. You're exhausted and have frequent headaches or stomachaches. Your resistance is low and you get sick more often. You're depressed. One particular sign to watch for is anger, especially when it's too frequent and too intense for the situation" (119).

There is growing interest in the strains experienced by those who care (emotionally and physically) for others who suffer. This is perhaps more noticeable as financial and political imperatives restructure the ways care is provided. The management of mental illness, disability, special needs, and palliative care is increasingly shrugged off by institutional or state providers, without compensatory development of support structures for the communities and individuals who take on the responsibility. Families are more dispersed, providing only frail networks of mutual assistance.

Venitia Sherson vividly describes the empathy required to be a nurse, the emotional strain of "giv[ing] endlessly," looking after exceptionally ill people day after day with little help or recognition. That the challenges of this often draining, sometimes rewarding, but always demanding devotion to others should be described in the idiom of disease is a commanding reminder of how diagnosis infuses how we make sense of our difficulties in Western society. "Compassion fatigue," "secondary victimization," "compassion contagion," "burnout syndrome," "countertransference," and "secondary traumatic stress disorder" are all used to describe the burden of caring (Sabo 2006). Compassion fatigue is referred to as a "condition," with victims, symptoms, screening tools, risk factors, and treatments. It has awareness projects, advocates, and perhaps one day will have its very own drugs.

The notion of "disorder" positions a particular experience (in this case, distress) as pathological or diseased (Horwitz 2007; Horwitz and Wakefield 2007). "Disorder" conveys a different meaning than "distress." Distress is the unhappy reaction that an individual might experience when faced with event—say, the death of a loved one, the loss of a job, or ill health. With distress, the reaction is to an external condition or a significant difficulty in daily life. As time goes on and the context improves, the individual should recover equilibrium, albeit not necessarily without sequelae or scars. Distress, one might say, is the normal reaction to an abnormal situation: how one would expect to feel when facing something intensely difficult. A disorder, on the contrary, is an abnormal response to either a normal or an abnormal situation. That is to say, it can be a reaction to something that should normally not cause distress, or it can exceed the range of typical reactions to the particular situation. A disordered distress is linked to an internal psychological dysfunction and is located within the individual rather than the social affront (Horwitz 2007).

Adams and colleagues' (2006) study provides a helpful example of how compassion fatigue has been cast as disorder, framed as a diagnosis. This study focuses on assessing a screening implement and its predictive validity for compassion fatigue. To do so, the researchers undertook a cross-sectional survey of social workers, chosen because of the high caseloads and low resourcing that characterize the field. Despite defining "compassion fatigue" as "the *natural* consequent behaviors and emotions resulting from knowing about a traumatizing event experienced or suffered by a person" (103, emphasis added)—a definition in line with the idea of distress rather than disorder—the study looks closely at characteristics of the *individual* to explain the cause. The authors consider what aspects of the health care provider's personal history and coping ability might explain or predict the development of compassion fatigue, looking at correlations between general health, stress, and psychological resources and the putative disorder. This situates the locus of the condition in the individual, shifting it from normal response to disorder.

Far from wishing to deny that those who bear heavy emotional burdens in caring for others may suffer, I would like nonetheless to propose alternative models for considering compassion fatigue. As mentioned above, Adams and colleagues (2006) focus on a dysfunction situated in the individual, trying to detect a frailty or predisposing factor for compassion fatigue. The authors see this work as a "prelude to devising intervention strategies designed to mitigate the negative effects on the care-giving practitioner" (108). The screening tool focuses firmly on the individual and opens the door for interventions within a disease model.

Conceptualizing compassion fatigue as a dysfunction of the individual rather than as a failure of the system closes off a number of other avenues for succor. An economic or political framing of this problem would not deny its existence but would situate its cause and remedy outside of the individual, in structural and political action. Had a labor, rather than a psychiatric, researcher decided to take on this study, they might have more intuitively chosen to look at workload and resourcing to understand in what circumstances one is more likely to feel distressed by helping traumatized or suffering individuals. Social policy and legislation may go further than individual treatment to eradicate what is probably less a "disorder" than a social problem.

But this is not terribly surprising. That the burden of compassion should be portrayed in terms of disease may also be a strategic mechanism to emphasize the importance of the challenge. Didier Fassin has spoken of how diagnoses bear witness to the world in authoritative ways. A diagnosis of PTSD brings credibility to subjective accounts of misery from those who have suffered natural disaster, war, or a combination of both. The diagnosis substitutes the words of the expert for the voice of the sufferer (Fassin 2009). In this sense diagnosis mediates suffering and translates it into terms that can no longer be ignored by national and international communities. The *DSM*-like, technocratic language of medicine compels action as it appropriates and transforms a narrative of human suffering to one of public health imperative.

The example of suffering depicted as disease underlines and epitomizes the social intrigue of diagnosis with which this book is concerned. Diagnosis tells us much about what we value and believe in as people; it behooves us to understand it well. Turner's (2007) and Shermis's (1962) work on new disciplines recommends that to anchor a field, one must consider and define what that field is and how it adds value to society's goals and aspirations. In response to these criteria, a sociology of diagnosis must be concerned with the creation, application, allocation, and exploitation of diagnostic categories.

Creation

What counts as disease and how is this determined? The classification of diseases and disease discovery processes is a rich source of study. Disease boundaries are ever shifting, as they negotiate where and how deviance becomes disease, feeling becomes symptom, and the stigmatized becomes value-free (Rosenberg 2006, 407). The development of diagnoses serves as an indication of what we are prepared to accept as normal, healthy, moral, and bearable. As new disease categories are recognized and incorporated into medicine's taxonomies, they draw together competing and concordant forces: lay activism can both buttress and dispute medical diagnosis.

Technology shifts diagnostic boundaries, just as education, resources, and social priorities shape technology's directions. Technology sees what is invisible to the naked eye. Elevated C-reactive protein, sickling cells, calcifications, and microfibrillary tangles indicate what sicknesses we may have. Whole-genome sequencing tells us what variant of corona- or influenza virus we are dealing with. The human genome project ultimately proposes a different way of classifying, relying on genetic susceptibility, until now unconsidered in the *ICD* and *DSM*.

Application

I have struggled throughout this text to find the *mot juste* to express the transfer of the diagnosis from the medical lexicon and the doctor's understanding of disease to the layperson's experience of illness. When the patient goes to the doctor, it is to await a kind of stamp or signet. Its mark determines what happens next, as the condition finds its expression in words that have meaning beyond the individual's perception. The experience of discomfort gets filed with the panoply of other experiences, which together make sense to a wider world. The layperson "gets diagnosed," a passive reidentification over which they have less control than they might like, and during which the person's illness becomes validated (or not). This is Blaxter's "process" of diagnosis (1978). Is a diagnosis conveyed? (No, too passive, too much like a property transaction.) Awarded? (Possibly, when having the label opens doors.) Branded? (When it's a stigmatizing diagnosis.) Applied? (Like trying on new lipstick.) Or disclosed? (When the severity and complexity of the condition requires a particular discretion and authority.)

Diagnosis is relational and strongly influenced by the positions occupied by doctor and layperson—sometimes on opposing, sometimes on supporting, sides. Anatole Broyard (1995) writes of his experience of diagnosis: "Just as he orders blood tests and bone scans of my body, I'd like my doctor to scan *me*, to grope for my spirit as well as my prostate. While he inevitably feels superior to me because he is the doctor and I am the patient, I'd like him to know that I feel superior to him too, that he is my patient also and I have my diagnosis of him. There should be a place where our respective superiorities could meet and frolic together" (179).

The changing roles that are played by lay and professional give pause. Freedom and autonomy, reliance and compliance, all parry and circle around the diagnosis and its application, conveyance, award, branding, or stamp.

Allocation

The diagnosis-resource link has threaded through this book, as it threads through the Western experience of disease. Parsons's (1958) early work on the sick role makes clear the first important resource: allowance. The diagnosis entitles the sick person to a different social expectation: the patient rests, misses work, gets help. It is the patient's due.

While I have cited both Freidson and de Swaan in reference to the power imbued in medicine, which serves as the gatekeeper of resources, I reprise their arguments here with a focus on diagnosis. They both knew that diagnosis was key in the allocation process. Recall that Freidson (1972) writes, "Where illness is the ubiquitous label for deviance in an age, the profession that is custodian of the label is ascendant" (244). De Swaan (1989) focuses on how, in the presence of scant resources, doctors are called on to make decisions about the distribution of goods such as housing, leave, insurance coverage, and treatment. Custodianship of the diagnostic label is shifting, as we can see from the changing lay-professional relationship, the mediatization of health, and the free flow of previously restricted-access medical information. But the diagnosis remains at the fulcrum of allocation.

Consider, for example, the authorization of particular medications, notably expensive ones. In many cases it is not enough for the doctor simply to diagnose and prescribe. Adalimumab is a case in point. Adalimumab is a monoclonal antibody that reduces the symptoms of ankylosing spondylitis, an inflammatory disease mainly affecting the spine, with often serious impact on daily function (McLeod et al. 2007). Given the high cost of this treatment, however, it is not given without formal diagnostic confirmation of serious ankylosing spondylitis. In New Zealand, for example, access to treatment by adalimumab is authorized only after a checklist of diagnostic criteria is submitted to the pharmaceutical management agency. The presence of sacroiliitis on X-rays and certain elevated nonspecific clinical markers (ESR and CRP) are prerequisites to treatment (Pharmac 2023). In this case and others like it, the doctor has a role in diagnosis but is powerless to override the administrative definition of the disease, whose standardized criteria fulfill the gatekeeping role. This speaks to what Turner describes as "the standardization of illness into phenomena which can be managed by bureaucratic agencies" (qtd. in Filc 2006).

Exploitation

Diagnoses provide fodder for exploitation: commercial, political, and personal. The "mongering" of diseases (Payer 1992) is not restricted to Big Pharma. The manufacturers of medical equipment, complementary and alternative therapies, nutritional supplements, and food products equally have an interest in promoting particular disease states. Television and media reap benefit from disease stories. Reality television features the fight against obesity (*The Biggest Loser, Weighing In, Celebrity Fit Club*); documentaries highlight personal battles against illness and disease education; self-help books, magazines, and infomercials often have disease as their focus. Gyms and fitness centers generate memberships on the basis of collective concern about obesity, hypertension, and other forms of cardiovascular disease.

Research teams are built around diseases, legitimate and contested, bringing private and public money along with students and high-profile staff to their institutions (Burgan 2005). Similarly, politicians are often willing to jump on disease bandwagons to identify with and exploit popular concerns.

At a personal level, there will be readers who miss work, calling in sick under the false pretext of a headache or influenza. Being sick is an acceptable reason for not going to work, whereas "getting the car registered before I get a ticket" is not. Taken to an extreme, malingering is the more severe exploitation of diagnostic status by an individual for personal benefit. Malingering implies fabricating symptoms to receive a diagnosis for some form of secondary gain. Not only might a malingerer shirk work or other social responsibilities; they might also pursue financial entitlements, medications, allowances, or simply attention that would otherwise not be permitted.

The fact that diagnoses can be exploited doesn't mean that any one diagnosis is more or less worthy than another, more or less "real." Rather, it reflects the power that putting a name to a condition generates. The fixed disease entity provides substance around which support and interest can rally and a range of agendas be met.

Directions for a Sociology of Diagnosis

I have been playing with Ockham's razor myself as I put this book together. I have attempted to look for patterns and boundaries in the study of disease, demonstrating what ideas might cogently be put together, what forces and effects are linked to one another, distinct from others and like enough to make sense to readers when placed in the same chapter. This process of classifying is the means by which we all make social sense of the world, making labels (words) that we can then use among ourselves to communicate our interests, hopes, and fears.

The important point, as Nick Fox and Katie Ward (2008) write, is that there is nothing prior and independent about health and disease. Rather, they are assemblages both borne of and acting to reconfirm relations and effects. Health and illness are political categories, they write, resulting just as much from "the physical and cultural possibilities and constraints *surrounding* a person's body as with any characteristic of the body itself" (1019, emphasis added).

A model for a sociology of diagnosis would inevitably need to consider disease as more than a given, a priori entity. This does not mean presuming that diagnostic categories are somehow neither real nor useful. Rather, it means considering how and why particular diseases are framed as they are and not in another way. It implies understanding the interest directed at some conditions as opposed to others and the desirability of some disease labels as contrasted with the unattractiveness of others.

The model depicted in figure 1 recognizes the assemblage that constitutes diagnosis, the relationality of the diagnostic moment, and the transformative potential of diagnosis as process. I do not propose the fragments that constitute the social framing and social consequences of diagnosis as absolute or complete categories. Reality is continuous, and deciding to lump or to split on the basis of an argument that I propose to my peers is a social action (Zerubavel 1996). It is convention, the same as that "which transforms actual oceans into mental archipelagos" (427). I have in this spirit created categories into which I am forcing reality with the fervor of the foregoing pages to convince my readers that my concept formation is sound.

I have modified the social model of diagnosis subtly since the previous edition. I snuck some words into what should have been called the "diagnostic process" (and wasn't) in the previous version. Of course this book is all about what Mildred Blaxter proposed in 1978, diagnosis-as-category, diagnosis-as-process, and, my add-on: social consequence.

Curiously, as I write these words today, I have a box of tissues at my side. I have what New Zealanders call a "lurgy." That's a word I had to learn after I moved here. It's not used in the United States. It's an unspecified illness: what my mother might have called "a bug." My own process as I experience this is to recognize the dysfunction and to curiously interrogate it. How do I really

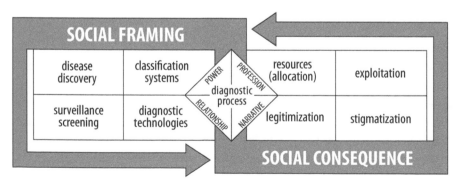

Figure 1. Social understanding of diagnosis (revised)

feel? Is there anything that worries me? Do my heart rate and temperature feel "normal"? I narrate my dysfunction, quietly to myself, think about the cold my grandson had, and settle with it. I don't think I need to get a name for it. It can stay a "lurgy" or a "bug." But then I hesitate, because I have access to a diagnostic tool I wouldn't have had when I drafted the first edition of this book. I pull out a rapid antigen test (we call them "RATs" in New Zealand) and check whether it's COVID-19. I care about one diagnosis but not about others. At the same time, being alone in the house for the week and not having to go to work, the consequence of not being diagnosed is minimal. I don't need treatment, I don't need resources, but I do have to have a way to talk about what I am experiencing. I don't want to tell everyone that I have a banal upper respiratory infection with a mild cough, runny nose, and scratchy throat. But I do have to reassure the electrician, when he comes by, that it's not COVID-19. That diagnosis would matter.

I have provided a second schema which shows how the model helps study and understand the COVID-19 diagnosis as a social phenomenon, a consensus, an agreement (figure 2). This applied version of the social model of diagnosis shows how we can implement sociological thinking about diagnosis.

I position this revised social model and the COVID-19 model as a renewed challenge to the discipline, encouraging its adherents to identify what elements help us understand diagnosis fully; how diagnosis influences and, in turn, is influenced by its social features; and what the pandemic has offered us as new avenues of reflection. A conversation on this subject is important to the field; as an emerging intellectual discipline, the sociology of diagnosis must have "techniques suitable for dealing with its concepts in order to develop a sus-

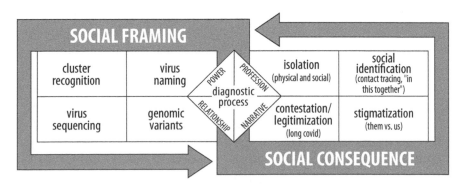

Figure 2. Social understanding of COVID-19

tainable intellectual tradition" (Shermis 1962, 84) and by extension, contribute to society's goals and aspirations (Turner 2007).

The social model of diagnosis (figure 1) illustrates how classifications are generated. Many forces and agents interact to create diagnoses and their consequences. These factors, however, are not independent in their own genesis, from their social consequence: it is a kind of chicken-and-egg situation. While diagnoses cannot import a social consequence until they become standardized as a label, the impact of the label continues to feed into the framing of diagnostic categories as they are, or as they will become. With each revision of the *Diagnostic and Statistical Manual of Mental Disorders* or of the *International Statistical Classification of Diseases and Related Health Problems*, there are drawn-out debates about how changing a diagnostic category will affect the treatment of a disease or the experience of those labeled with it, or about how current categories either achieve or fail to fulfill their promise. I have explored how lay movements, as well as commercial exploitation, have fed into the social framing of diagnostic categories. On the one hand, in the case of homosexuality, stigmatization drove the movement to change its diagnostic status. On the other hand, the drive for recognition of female hypoactive sexual desire disorder is largely driven by pharmaceutical industry interests.

But this is not a one-way model. Just as the social consequences of diagnosis mold the disease classifications, so do the classifications frame the experiences of diagnosis, a point that hardly needs amplification. As one example, state employees of Alabama have been compelled since 2009 to subject themselves to an annual medical examination including the measurement of BMI. Those who are subsequently diagnosed as obese face an increased insurance premium (Fernandez 2008). This diagnosis results in immediate financial consequences. In contrast, diagnosis and impairment ratings are at the heart of disability determination in the case of fibromyalgia and other illness that result in work incapacity (Hadler 1996). An individual seeking disability payments would see the diagnosis as key in their pursuit.

In both cases, the consequences of the diagnosis (stigmatization for the obese and resources for those with fibromyalgia) feed into the circular relationship described above. Patient advocacy groups, researchers, and insurers will all have their ideas about how better to frame the problems of chronic fatigue or obesity.

The dynamic social nature of diagnosis and the diagnostic process is an important point of academic reflection precisely because diagnoses are not prior ontological entities but social categories that organize, direct, explain, and sometimes control our experience of health and illness. Bowker and Star (1999) describe classifications as a kind of "work practice" but an invisible one, valorizing some points of view and silencing others (50). The inevitable privileging of certain voices over others in medical classification is opaque and must be made visible. The model proposed above for the sociological analysis of diagnosis provides a tool for revealing the points of view that are contained in a disease label. Importantly, reminds Weinberg (2020), disease categories are not "immune to the explanatory repertoire of sociology" (2).

The power of sociological analysis is its potential to reveal the deep layers of negotiation, compromise, and interests that cover and surround the scientific evidence of a disease. The assemblages and boundaries that circumscribe disease often have an untapped elasticity that social inquiry can both challenge and reconfigure.

References

Aalton, C. M., M. M. Samson, and P. A. F. Jansen. 2006. Diagnostic errors: The need to have autopsies. *Netherlands Journal of Medicine* 64 (6):186–90.

Abenhaim, Lucien, Michel Rossignol, Jean-Pierre Valat, Margareta Nordin, Bernard Avouac, Francis Blotman, Jacques Charlot, Renee Liliane Dreiser, Erick Legrand, Sylvie Rozenberg, and Philippe Vautravers. 2000. The role of activity in the therapeutic management of back pain: Report of the International Paris Task Force on Back Pain. *Spine* 24 (4S):1S–33S.

Abraham, John. 2007. Building on sociological understandings of the pharmaceutical industry or reinventing the wheel? Response to Joan Busfield, Pills, power, people. *Sociology* 41 (4):727–36.

Adams, R. E., J. A. Boscarino, and C. R. Figley. 2006. Compassion fatigue and psychological distress among social workers: A validation study. *American Journal of Orthopsychiatry* 76 (1):103–8.

Album, D., L. E. Johannessen, and E. B. Rasmussen. 2017. Stability and change in disease prestige: A comparative analysis of three surveys spanning a quarter of a century. *Social Science and Medicine* 180:45–51. https://doi.org/10.1016/j.socscimed.2017.03.020.

Album, D., and S. Westin. 2008. Do diseases have a prestige hierarchy? A survey among physicians and medical students. *Social Science and Medicine* 66 (1):182–88. https://doi.org/10.1016/j.socscimed.2007.07.003.

Alexander, Archie. 2007. "Just scanning around" with diagnostic medical ultrasound: Should states regulate the non-diagnostic use of this technology? *Annals of Health Law* 16 (1):1–42.

Amaducci, Luigi. A., Walter. A. Rocca, and Bruce. S. Schoenberg. 1986. Origin of the distinction between Alzheimer's disease and senile dementia: How history can clarify nosology. *Neurology* 36 (11):1497–99.

American Pregnancy Association. 2023. Keepsake ultrasounds. https://americanpregnancy.org/healthy-pregnancy/pregnancy-health-wellness/keepsake-ultrasound/.

American Psychiatric Association (APA). 2000. Generalized anxiety disorder. In *Diagnostic and Statistical Manual of Mental Disorders* (4th ed., text revisions). Washington, DC: American Psychiatric Association.

Apple, Rima D. 1995. Constructing mothers: Scientific motherhood in the nineteenth and twentieth centuries. *Social History of Medicine* 8 (2):161–78.

Arbeitskreis Blut, U. B. B. K. 2009. Influenza virus. *Transfusion Medicine and Hemotherapy: Offizielles Organ der Deutschen Gesellschaft fur Transfusionsmedizin und Immunhamatologie* 36:32–39.

Armstrong, David. 1995. The rise of surveillance medicine. *Sociology of Health and Illness* 17 (3):393–404.

Arnold, Thomas. 1839. *On the Divisions and Mutual Relations of Knowledge: A Lecture Read before the Rugby Literary and Scientific Society, April 7, 1835.* Rugby, UK: Combe and Crossley.

Arnow, Bruce A., Enid Hunkeler, Christine Blasey, Janelle Lee, Michael Constantino, Bruce Fireman, Helena Kraemer, Robin Dea, Rebecca Robinson, and Chris Hayward. 2006. Comorbid depression, chronic pain, and disability in primary care. *Psychosomatic Medicine* 68 (2):262–68.

Aronowitz, Robert. 1998. *Making Sense of Illness: Science, Society, and Disease.* Cambridge: Cambridge University Press.

Aronowitz, Robert. 2001. When do symptoms become a disease? *Annals of Internal Medicine* 134 (9 part 2):803–8.

Aronowitz, Robert. 2008. Framing disease: An underappreciated mechanism for the social patterning of health. *Social Science and Medicine* 67 (1):1–9.

Augustine. 1990. *Sermons II.* Translated by E. Hill. New York: New City Press.

Ayer's Sarsaparilla. 1896. Beauty begins in the blood. *Godey's*, January, 115.

Balint, Michael. 1964. *The Doctor, His Patient and the Illness* (2nd ed.). Kent, UK: Pitman Medical.

Ban, Thomas. A. 2006. The role of serendipity in drug discovery. *Dialogues in Clinical Neuroscience* 8 (3):335–44.

Barker, Kristin K. 1998. A ship upon a stormy sea: The medicalization of pregnancy. *Social Science and Medicine* 47 (8):1067–76.

Barker, Kristin, and Tasha R. Galardi. 2015. Diagnostic domain defense: Autism spectrum disorder and the *DSM-5. Social Problems* 62 (1):120–40.

Barsky, Arthur J., and Jonathan F. Borus. 1999. Functional somatic syndromes. *Annals of Internal Medicine* 130 (11):910–21.

Basson, Rosemary, Jennifer Berman, Arthur Burnett, Leonard Derogatis, David Ferguson, Jean Fourcroy, Irwin Goldstein, Allesandra Graziottin, Julia Heiman, Ellen Laan, et al. 2000. Report of the International Consensus Development Conference on Female Sexual Dysfunction: Definitions and classifications. *Journal of Urology* 163 (3):888–93.

Becker, Gay, and Robert D. Nachtigall. 1992. Eager for medicalisation: The social production of infertility as a disease. *Sociology of Health and Illness* 14 (4):456–71.

Berger, Peter L., and Thomas Luckmann. 1966. *The Social Construction of Reality: A Treatise in the Sociology of Knowledge.* Garden City, NY: Doubleday.

Berlin, Leonard, and Jonathan W. Berlin. 2005. Leasing imaging facilities to referring physicians: Fee shifting or fee splitting? *Radiology* 234 (1):44–48.

Bertillon, Jacques. 1909. *Nomenclatures des maladies: Statistique de morbidité—statistique des causes de décès.* Paris: Montevrain.

Best, J. (Ed.). 1989. *Images of Issues: Typifying Contemporary Social Problems*. Hawthorne, NY: Aldine de Gruyter.

Billig, M. 1995. *Banal Nationalism*. London: Sage.

Black, William C. 2000. Overdiagnosis: An underrecognized cause of confusion and harm in cancer screening. *Journal of the National Cancer Institute* 92 (16): 1280–82.

Blaxter, Mildred. 1978. Diagnosis as category and process: The case of alcoholism. *Social Science and Medicine* 12:9–17.

Blaxter, Mildred. 2009. The case of the vanishing patient? Image and experience. *Sociology of Health and Illness* 31 (5):762–78.

Boehringer Ingelheim (BI). 2008. Hypoactive sexual desire disorder backgrounder. *Boehringer Ingelheim Science and Technology Communications*, May.

Bogaert, Anthony F. 2004. Asexuality: Prevalence and associated factors in a national probability sample. *Journal of Sex Research* 41 (3):279–87.

Bonnie, Richard J. 2002. Political abuse of psychiatry in the Soviet Union and in China: Complexities and controversies. *Journal of the American Academy of Psychiatry and the Law* 30:136–44.

Booth, Eric W. 1991. Compassion fatigue. *Journal of the American Medical Association* 266 (3):362.

Borsini, F., R. Cesana, J. Kelly, B. E. Leonard, M. McNamara, J. Richards, and L. Seiden. 1997. BIMT-17: A putative antidepressant with a fast onset of action? *Psychopharmacology* 134 (4):378–86.

Borsini, Franco, and Kenneth R. Evans. 2006. Method of treating female hypoactive sexual desire disorder with Flibanserin. US patent 7151103 (10/272603).

Borsini, Franco, E. Giraldo, E. Monferini, G. Antonini, M. Parenti, G. Bietti, and A. Donetti. 1995. BIMT-17, a 5-HT2A receptor antagonist and 5-HT1A receptor full agonist in rat cerebral cortex. *Naunyn-Schmiedebergs Archives of Pharmacology* 352 (3):276–82.

Bove, A. A. 2008. Internet-based medical education. *Perspectives in Biology and Medicine* 51 (1):61–70.

Bowker, Geoffrey C. 1996. The history of information infrastructures: The case of the international classification of diseases. *Information Processing and Management* 32 (1):49–61.

Bowker, Geoffrey C., and Susan Leigh Star. 1999. *Sorting Things Out: Classification and Its Consequences*. Cambridge, MA: MIT Press.

Bowker, Geoffrey C., and Susan Leigh Star. 2000. Invisible mediators of action: Classification and the ubiquity of standards. *Mind, Culture, and Activity* 7 (1):147–63.

Brackenbury, H. 1934. Patient and doctor. *British Medical Journal* 2:205–8.

Brady, Anita. 2007. "Constituting Queer: Performativity and Commodity Culture, Media Studies." PhD diss., University of Otago, Dunedin.

Bricart, Isabelle. 1985. *Saintes ou pouliches: L'éducation des jeunes filles au XIXème siècle*. Paris: Albion Michel.

British Medical Journal. 1886. The nomenclature of medicine. 1 (1328):1114–28.

172   *References*

Brody, Howard. 2006. Informed refusal. *Virtual Mentor* 8 (1):24–29.

Brown, David Allen. 2001. *Virtue and Beauty: Leonardo's "Ginevra de' Benci" and Renaissance Portraits of Women*. Princeton, NJ: Princeton University Press.

Brown, Phil. 1990. The name game: Toward a sociology of diagnosis. *Journal of Mind and Behaviour* 11 (3/4):385–406.

Brown, Phil. 1995. Naming and framing: the social construction of diagnosis and illness. *Journal of Health and Social Behavior* (Health Module):34–52.

Brown, Phil. 2008. Naming and framing: The social construction of diagnosis and illness. In *Perspectives in Medical Sociology*, edited by P. Brown. Long Grove, IL: Waveland Press.

Brown, Phil, and Stephen Zavestoski. 2004. Social movements in health: An introduction. *Sociology of Health and Illness* 26 (6):679–94.

Brown, Phil, Stephen Zavestoski, Sabrina McCormick, Brian Mayer, Rachel Morello-Frosch, and Rebecca Gasior Altman. 2004. Embodied health movements: New approaches to social movements in health. *Sociology of Health and Illness* 26 (1):50–80.

Broyard, Anatole. 1995. Doctor, talk to me. In *On Doctoring*, edited by R. Reynolds and J. Stone. New York: Simon and Schuster.

Brubaker, S. J., and H. E. Dillaway. 2009. Medicalization, natural childbirth and birthing experiences. *Sociology Compass* 3:31–48.

Buetow, Stephen A. 2005. To care is to coprovide. *Annals of Family Medicine* 3 (6): 553–55.

Buetow, Stephen A., Annemarie Jutel, and Karen Hoare. 2009. Shrinking social space in the doctor–modern patient relationship: A review of forces for, and implications of, homologization. *Patient Education and Counseling* 74 (1):97–103.

Burgan, Mary. 2005. Superstars and rookies of the year: Faculty hiring practices in the post-modern age. Center for Studies in Higher Education Research and Occasional Papers Series CSHE.10.05:1–17.

Burr, Vivien. 1995. *An Introduction to Social Constructionism*. London: Routledge.

Busfield, Joan. 2006. Pills, power, people: Sociological understandings of the pharmaceutical industry. *Sociology* 40 (2):297–314.

Busfield, Joan, and Jo Campling. 1996. *Men, Women, and Madness: Understanding Gender and Mental Disorder*. Washington Square: New York University Press.

California Fig Syrup. 1896. Syrup of figs. *Godey's*, January, back cover.

Callard, Felicity, and Elisa Perego. 2021. How and why patients made Long Covid. *Social Science and Medicine* 268:113426. https://doi.org/10.1016/j.socscimed.2020.113426.

Campos, Paul, Abigail Saguy, Paul Ernsberger, Eric Oliver, and Glenn Gaesser. 2006. The epidemiology of overweight and obesity: Public health crisis or moral panic? *International Journal of Epidemiology* 35 (1):55–60.

Carey, John. 2006. Viagra for women? *Businessweek*, December 28. https://www.bloomberg.com/news/articles/2006-12-28/viagra-for-women-businessweek-business-news-stock-market-and-financial-advice.

Cartwright, Samuel A. 1981. Report of the diseases and physical peculiarities of the Negro race. In *Concepts of Health and Disease*, edited by A. Caplan, H. T. Englehardt, and J. McCartney. Reading, MA: Addison-Wesley. Also available online at https://www.pbs.org/wgbh/aia/part4/4h3106t.html.

Carver, Raymond. 1998. What the doctor said. In *All of Us: The Collected Poems*. New York: Knopf.

Cassell, Eric J. 1991. *The Nature of Suffering and the Goals of Medicine*. New York: Oxford University Press.

Cassidy, J. 1991. Compassion fatigue: Healthcare professionals are vulnerable as care giving becomes more stressful. *Health Progress* 72 (1):54–55, 64.

Caux, Chantal, David J. Roy, Louise Guilbert, and Claude Viau. 2007. Anticipating ethical aspects of the use of biomarkers in the workplace: A tool for stakeholders. *Social Science and Medicine* 65 (2):344–54.

CDC (Centers for Disease Control and Prevention). 2008. Avian influenza A virus infections of humans. http://www.cdc.gov/flu/avian/gen-info/avian-flu-humans.htm.

CDC (Centers for Disease Control and Prevention). 2009a. Interim guidance on infection control measures for 2009 H1N1 influenza in healthcare settings, including protection of healthcare personnel. www.cdc.gov/h1n1flu/guidelines_infection _control.htm. Accessed November 16, 2009.

CDC (Centers for Disease Control and Prevention). 2009b. *Morbidity and Mortality Weekly Report* 58 (15), April 24.

CDC (Centers for Disease Control and Prevention). 2012. An introduction to applied epidemiology and biostatistics. *Principles of Epidemiology in Public Health Practice*, 3rd ed. Atlanta: US Department of Health and Human Services.

CDC (Centers for Disease Control and Prevention). 2022. Life expectancy in the U.S. dropped for the second year in a row in 2021. National Center for Health Statistics, August 31.

CDC (Centers for Disease Control and Prevention). 2023. About overweight and obesity. https://www.cdc.gov/obesity/about-obesity/index.html. Accessed November 28, 2023.

Charland, Louis C. 2004. A madness for identity: Psychiatric labels, consumer autonomy, and the perils of the Internet. *Philosophy, Psychiatry, and Psychology* 11 (4):336–49.

Chaufan, C., B. Hollister, J. Nazareno, and P. Fox. 2012. Medical ideology as a double-edged sword: The politics of cure and care in the making of Alzheimer's disease. *Social Science and Medicine* 74 (5):788–95. https://doi.org/10.1016/j.socscimed.2011 .10.033.

Chen, J. S. 2021. What is in a name? Autonomic imbalance and medically unexplained symptoms in Taiwan. *Sociology of Health and Illness* 43:881–94. https://on linelibrary.wiley.com/doi/10.1111/1467-9566.13262.

Cheng, D. 2020. Covid 19 coronavirus: What alert level 3 and other levels mean for you. *New Zealand Herald*, April 16. https://www.nzherald.co.nz/nz/news/article .cfm?c_id=1&objectid=12325179.

Chiri, G., M. Bergey, and T. I. Mackie. 2022. Deserving but not entitled: The social construction of autism spectrum disorder in federal policy. *Social Science and Medicine* 301:114974. https://doi.org/10.1016/j.socscimed.2022.114974.

Christie, William F. 1927. *Surplus Fat and How to Reduce It*. London: Heinemann/ Medical Books.

Clark, Jack A., and Elliot Mishler, G. 1992. Attending to patients' stories: Reframing the clinical task. *Sociology of Health and Illness* 14 (3):344–72.

Clarke, Adele E., and Monica J. Casper. 1996. From simple technology to complex arena: Classification of pap smears, 1917–90. *Medical Anthropology Quarterly* 10 (4):601–23.

Clarke, Adele E., Janet K. Shim, Laura Mamo, Jennifer Ruth Fosket, and Jennifer R. Fishman. 2003. Biomedicalization: Technoscientific transformations of health, illness, and U.S. biomedicine. *American Sociological Review* 68 (2):161–94.

Clayton, Anita H., Evan R. Goldfischer, Irwin Goldstein, Leonard Derogatis, Diane J. Lewis-D'Agostino, and Robert Pyke. 2009. Validation of the decreased sexual desire screener (DSDS): A brief diagnostic instrument for generalized acquired female hypoactive sexual desire disorder (HSDD). *Journal of Sexual Medicine* 6 (3):730–38.

Cochrane, Archie L. 1989. Archie Cochrane in his own words. Selections arranged from his 1972 introduction to *Effectiveness and Efficiency: Random Reflections on the Health Services. Control Clinical Trials* 10 (4):428–33.

Cohen, Marc S. 2008. Aristotle's *Metaphysics*. In *Stanford Encyclopedia of Philosophy*, edited by E. N. Zalta. Stanford, CA: Metaphysics Research Lab. plato.stanford .edu/entries/aristotle-metaphysics/#Cat.

Cohen, Stanley. 1980. *Folk Devils and Moral Panics: The Creation of the Mods and Rockers*. New York: St. Martin's Press.

Conrad, Kathryn. 2001. Foetal Ireland: National bodies and political agency. *Eire-Ireland*, Fall/Winter:157–73.

Conrad, Peter. 1975. The discovery of hyperkinesis: Notes on the medicalization of deviant behavior. *Social Problems* 23 (1):12–21.

Conrad, Peter. 1979. Types of medical social control. *Sociology of Health and Illness* 1 (1):1–11.

Conrad, Peter. 1992. Medicalization and social control. *Annual Review of Sociology* 18:209–32.

Conrad, Peter. 2005. The shifting engines of medicalization. *Journal of Health and Social Behavior* 46 (1):3–14.

Conrad, Peter. 2007. *The Medicalization of Society: On the Transformation of Human Conditions into Treatable Disorders*. Baltimore: Johns Hopkins University Press.

Conrad, Peter, and Valerie Leiter. 2004. Medicalization, markets and consumers. *Journal of Health and Social Behavior* 45 (Suppl.):158–76.

Conrad, Peter, and Joseph W. Schneider. 1980. *Deviance and Medicalization: From Badness to Sickness*. St. Louis: C. V. Mosby.

Corbett, Kevin, and Tristen Westwood. 2005. "Dangerous and severe personality disorder": A psychiatric manifestation of the risk society. *Critical Public Health* 15 (2):121–33.

Coughlan, T. 2020. Coronavirus: Chris Hipkins and Ashley Bloomfield slam spreading of "vile" rumours about latest Covid-19 cluster. *Stuff*, August 16. https://www .stuff.co.nz/national/health/coronavirus/300083605/coronavirus-chris-hipkins -and-ashley-bloomfield-slam-spreading-of-vile-rumours-about-latest-covid19-cluster.

Cowan, L., and M. Wainwright. 2001. The death of a baby in our care: The impact on the midwife. *Midwifery Digest* 11 (3):313–16.

Crenner, C. 2005. *Private Practice in the Early Twentieth-Century Medical Office of Dr. Richard Cabot*. Baltimore: Johns Hopkins University Press.

Croskerry, Pat. 2002. Achieving quality in clinical decision making: Cognitive strategies and detection of bias. *Academic Emergency Medicine* 9 (11):1184–205.

Cushman, Philip. 1990. Why the self is empty: Toward a historically situated psychology. *American Psychologist* 45 (5):599–611.

Daniel, Thomas M. 2006. The history of tuberculosis. *Respiratory Medicine* 100 (11):1862–70.

Davis, G. 2015. *Contesting intersex: The dubious diagnosis*. New York: New York University Press.

Deale, Alicia, and Simon Wessely. 2001. Patients' perceptions of medical care in chronic fatigue syndrome. *Social Science and Medicine* 52 (12):1859–64.

Dear, James W., and David J. Webb. 2007. Disease mongering: A challenge for everyone involved in healthcare. *British Journal of Clinical Pharmacology* 64 (2):122–24.

Derogatis, Leonard R., Raymond Rosen, Sandra Leiblum, Arthur Burnett, and Julia Heiman. 2002. The female sexual distress scale (FSDS): Initial validation of a standardized scale for assessment of sexually related personal distress in women. *Journal of Sex and Marital Therapy* 28 (4):317–30.

de Boer, Marjolein Lotte, and Jenny Slatman. 2023. Producing Me/Cfs in Dutch newspapers: A social-discursive analysis about non/credibility. *Social Epistemology* 37 (5):592–609. https://doi.org/10.1080/02691728.2023.2171748.

de Swaan, Abram. 1989. The reluctant imperialism of the medical profession. *Social Science and Medicine* 28 (11):1165–70.

Dewhurst, Kenneth. 1966. *Dr. Thomas Sydenham, 1624–1689: His Life and Original Writings*. Berkeley: University of California Press.

Dietary Guidelines Advisory Committee. 1995. *Report of the Dietary Guidelines Advisory Committee on the Dietary Guidelines for Americans*. Washington, DC: United States Department of Agriculture.

Dinos, S., S. Stevens, M. Serfaty, S. Weich, and M. King. 2004. Stigma: The feelings and experiences of 46 people with mental illness. *British Journal of Psychiatry* 184:176–81.

Dixon, Jane, and Cathy Banwell. 2004. Re-embedding trust: Unravelling the construction of modern diets. *Critical Public Health* 14 (2):117–31.

Do I have ME/CFS? 2022. Online quiz. https://solvecfs.org/me-cfs-long-covid/do-i -have-mecfs-quiz/. Accessed June 6, 2023.

Drug and Therapeutics Bulletin. 2009. Testosterone patches for female sexual dysfunction. *Drug and Therapeutics Bulletin* 47:30–34. https://doi.org/10.1136/dtb.2009.02.0007.

Dumit, Joseph. 2006. Illnesses you have to fight to get: Facts as forces in uncertain, emergent illnesses. *Social Science and Medicine* 62 (3):577–90.

Durham, John. 2002. Population screening for prostate cancer: A systematic review. In *New Zealand Guidelines Group*. Wellington, NZ: University of Otago Department of General Practice.

Durkheim, Emile, and Marcel Mauss. 1903. De quelques formes de classification: Contribution à l'étude des représentations collectives. *Année sociologique* 6:1–72.

Elran-Barak, Roni, and Yoav Bar-Anan. 2018. Implicit and explicit anti-fat bias: The role of weight-related attitudes and beliefs. *Social Science and Medicine* 204:117–24. https://doi.org/10.1016/j.socscimed.2018.03.018.

Emanuel, Ezekiel J., and Linda L. Emanuel. 1992. Four models of the physician-patient relationship. *Journal of the American Medical Association* 267 (16):2221–26.

Engelhardt, H. Tristram. 1992. The body as a field of meaning: Implications for the ethics of diagnosis. In *The Ethics of Diagnosis*, edited by J. L. Peset and D. Gracia. Dordrecht: Kluwer Academic.

Epstein, Steven. 1996. *Impure Science: AIDS, Activism, and the Politics of Knowledge*. Berkeley: University of California Press.

Erlbeck, Hana H. 2001. *The Legends of the Demi-god Maui-Tikitiki-a-Taranga*. Auckland, NZ: Reed.

Evidence-Based Medicine Working Group. 1992. Evidence-based medicine: A new approach to teaching the practice of medicine. *Journal of the American Medical Association* 268 (17):2420–25.

Facing Our Risk. 2008. Previvor: Past, Present, and Future. Blog post. https://facingourrisk.wordpress.com/2008/07/22/previvor-past-present-future/.

Fassin, Didier. 2009. Global public health. In *Medical Anthropology at the Intersections: Celebrating 50 Years of Interdisciplinarity*. New Haven, CT: Yale University Press.

FDA (Food and Drug Administration). 2015. Center for Drug Evaluation and Research and Research Application Number 022526Orig1000. Medical review(s), August 17. http://www.accessdata.fda.gov/drugsatfda_docs/nda/2015/022526Orig1000MedR.pdf.

Feldman, Simon D., and Alfred I. Tauber. 1997. Sickle cell anemia: Reexamining the first "molecular disease." *Bulletin of the History of Medicine* 71 (4):623–50.

Fernandez, Don. 2008. Alabama "obesity penalty" stirs debate. CBS News Health, August 25. https://www.cbsnews.com/news/alabama-obesity-penalty-stirs-debate/.

Fenton, J. J., M. S. Weyrich, S. Durbin, Y. Liu, H. Bang, and J. Melnikow. 2018. *Prostate-specific antigen-based screening for prostate cancer: A systematic evidence review for the U.S. Preventive Services Task Force [Internet]*. May. Report No.: 17-05229-EF-1. Rockville, MD: Agency for Healthcare Research and Quality (US). PMID: 30085502.

Ferris, D. G., C. Dekle, and M. S. Litaker. 1996. Women's use of over-the-counter antifungal medications for gynecologic symptoms. *Journal of Family Practice* 42 (6):595–600.

Ferris, D. G., P. Nyirjesy, J. D. Sobel, D. Soper, A. Pavletic, and M. S. Litaker. 2002. Over-the-counter antifungal drug misuse associated with patient-diagnosed vulvovaginal candidiasis. *Obstetrics and Gynecology* 99 (3):419–25.

Filc, Dani. 2006. Power in the primary care medical encounter: Domination, resistance and alliances. *Social Theory and Health* 4:221–43.

Firebaugh, Glenn. 2015. Ecological fallacy, statistics of. In *International Encyclopedia of the Social and Behavioral Sciences*, 2nd ed., edited by James D. Wright. Amsterdam: Elsevier.

Fischer-Homberger, Esther. 1970. Eighteenth-century nosology and its survivors. *Medical History* 14 (4):397–403.

Flegal, Katherine M. 2006. Commentary: The epidemic of obesity; What's in a name? *International Journal of Epidemiology* 35 (1):72–74, discussion on 81–82.

Flegal, Katherine M., Barry I. Graubard, David. F. Williamson, and Mitchell H. Gail. 2005. Excess deaths associated with underweight, overweight, and obesity. *Journal of the American Medical Association* 293 (15):1861–67.

Fleischman, Suzanne. 1999. I am . . . , I have . . . , I suffer from . . . : A linguist reflects on the language of illness and disease. *Journal of Medical Humanities* 20 (1):1–31.

Fleiss, Joseph L., William Lawlor, Stanley R. Platman, and Ronald R. Fieve. 1971. On the use of inverted factor analysis for generating typologies. *Journal of Abnormal Psychology* 77 (2):127–32.

Foucar, Elliot. 2001. Classification in anatomic pathology. *American Journal of Clinical Pathology* 116 (Suppl.):S5–S20.

Foucault, Michel. 1963. *Naissance de la clinique*. Paris: Presses Universitaires de France.

Fox, Nick, and Katie Ward. 2006. Health identities: From expert patient to resisting consumer. *Health* (London) 10 (4):461–79.

Fox, Nick, and Katie Ward. 2008. What are health identities and how may we study them? *Sociology of Health and Illness* 30 (7):1007–21.

Fox, Nick, Katie Ward, and Alan O'Rourke. 2005. Pro-anorexia, weight-loss drugs and the internet: An "anti-recovery" explanatory model of anorexia. *Sociology of Health and Illness* 27 (7):944–71.

Fox, Patrick. 1989. From senility to Alzheimer's disease: The rise of the Alzheimer's disease movement. *Milbank Quarterly* 67 (1):58–102.

Frances, A. 2010. Opening Pandora's box: The 19 worst suggestions for *DSM-5*. *Psychiatric Times* 27 (3). https://go.gale.com/ps/i.do?p=AONE&u=googlescholar&id=GALE|A221434272&v=2.1&it=r&sid=AONE&asid=a3f377d3.

Frank, Arthur W. 1995. *The Wounded Storyteller: Body, Illness, and Ethics*. Chicago: University of Chicago Press.

Frayon, S., S. Cherrier, Y. Cavaloc, G. Wattelez, Y. Lerrant, and O. Galy. 2018. Relationship of body fat and body mass index in young Pacific Islanders: A cross-sectional study in European, Melanesian and Polynesian groups. *Pediatric Obesity* 13 (6):357–64. https://doi.org/10.1111/ijpo.12229. Epub July 28, 2017. PMID: 28752614.

Freemantle, Nick, and Mel Calvert. 2007. Composite and surrogate outcomes in randomised controlled trials. *British Medical Journal* (334):756–57.

Freidson, Eliot. 1972. *Profession of Medicine: A Study of the Sociology of Applied Knowledge*. 4th printing ed. New York: Dodd, Mead.

Furedi, Frank. 2006. The end of professional dominance. *Society* 43 (6):14–18.

Gaesser, Glenn A. 1999. Has body weight become an unhealthy obsession? *Medicine and Science in Sports and Exercise* 31:1118–28.

Gaines, Atwood D. 1992. From *DSM-I* to *III-R*; voices of self, mastery and the other: A cultural constructivist reading of U.S. psychiatric classification. *Social Science and Medicine* 35 (1):3–24.

Galdas, Paul M., Francine Cheater, and Paul Marshall. 2005. Men and help-seeking behaviour: Literature review. *Journal of Advanced Nursing* 6:616–23.

Gallo, Robert C., and Luc Montagnier. 2003. The discovery of HIV as the cause of AIDS. *New England Journal of Medicine* 349 (24):2283–85.

Gardener, A. 2019. A *Times* column, now streaming. *New York Times*, April 16:2. https://www.nytimes.com/2019/08/16/reader-center/diagnosis-tv-netflix.html.

Gellad, W. F., K. E. Flynn, and G. C. Alexander. 2015. Evaluation of flibanserin: Science and advocacy at the FDA. *JAMA* 314 (9):869–70. https://doi.org/10.1001/jama.2015.8405.

Gersuny, R. 1889. *Doctor and Patient: Hints to Both*. Bristol: John Wright.

Getz, Linn, Johann A. Sigurdsson, Irene Hetlevik, Anna L. Kirkengen, Solfrid Romundstad, and Jostein Holmen. 2005. Estimating the high risk group for cardiovascular disease in the Norwegian HUNT 2 population according to the 2003 European guidelines: Modelling study. *British Medical Journal* 331 (7516):551.

Gevitz, Norman. 2000. "The devil hath laughed at the physicians": Witchcraft and medical practice in seventeenth-century New England. *Journal of the History of Medicine* 55 (1):5–36.

Gilman, Sander L. 1991. *The Jew's Body*. New York: Routledge.

Goldstein, Annemarie. 2007. Medicine's flight from interpretation: When a cough is simply a cough. *Clinical Ethics* 2 (1):15–18.

Goldstein, Dianne E. 2004. Communities of suffering and the internet. In *Emerging Illnesses and Society: Negotiating the Public Health Agenda*, edited by R. M. Packard, P. J. Brown, R. L. Berkelman and H. Frumkin. Baltimore: Johns Hopkins University Press.

Goode, Erich. 1969. Marijuana and the politics of reality. *Journal of Health and Social Behavior* 10 (2):83–94.

Gough, Christina. 2023. Gym, health and fitness club industry revenue in the United States 2012–2023. Statista. https://www.statista.com/statistics/605223/us-fitness-health-club-market-size-2007-2021/. Accessed November 29, 2023.

Government of Canada. 2020. *Coronavirus disease (COVID-19)*. Modified June 19, 2023. https://www.canada.ca/en/public-health/services/diseases/coronavirus-disease-covid-19.html. Accessed October 3, 2020.

Government of Ireland. 2020. Taoiseach launches #InThisTogether campaign for people to stay connected, stay active and stay mentally well during COVID-19. https://www.gov.ie/en/press-release/433dof-an-taoiseach-launches-inthistogether -campaign-for-people-to-stay-con/. Accessed December 14, 2023.

Graber, Mark, Ruthanna Gordon, and Nancy Franklin. 2002. Reducing diagnostic errors in medicine: What's the goal? *Academic Medicine* 77 (10):981–92.

Graunt, John. 1662a. *Natural and Political Observations, Mentionned in a following Index, and made upon the Bills of Mortality.* London: John Martin, James Allestry, and the Dicas.

Graunt, John. 1662b. *Reflections on the Weekly Bills of Mortality for the Cities of London and Westminster and the Places adjacent but more especially, so far as it relates to the Plague and other Most Moral Diseases that we English-men are most subject to, and should be most careful against in this our age.* London: Samuel Speed.

Grimes, David A., and Kenneth F. Schulz. 2005. Surrogate end points in clinical research: Hazardous to your health. *Obstetrics and Gynecology* 105 (5 [part 1]):1114–18.

Gurwitz, Jerry H., Thomas J. McLaughlin, and Leslie S. Fish. 1995. The effect of an Rx-to-OTC switch on medication prescribing patterns and utilization of physician services: The case of vaginal antifungal products. *Health Services Research* 30 (5):672–85.

Hacking, Ian. 2001. Inaugural lecture: Chair of philosophy and history of scientific concepts at the Collège de France, January 16, 2001. *Economy and Society* 31 (1):1–14.

Hadler, Nortin M. 1996. If you have to prove you are ill, you can't get well: The object lesson of fibromyalgia. *Spine* 21 (20):2397–400.

Han, Paul K. 1997. Historical changes in the objectives of the periodic health examination. *Annals of Internal Medicine* 127 (10):910–17.

Hanna, E., and B. Gough. 2020. The social construction of male infertility: A qualitative questionnaire study of men with a male factor infertility diagnosis. *Sociology of Health and Illness* 42:465–480.

Hanne, M., and S. J. Hawken. 2007. Metaphors for illness in contemporary media. *Medical Humanities* 33:93–99.

Harrington, Patricia, and Marvin D. Shepherd. 2002. Analysis of the movement of prescription drugs to over-the-counter status. *Journal of Managed Care Pharmacy* 8 (6):499–508, quiz on 509–11.

Hayes, Brett, and Roger Adams. 2008. Parallels between clinical reasoning and categorization. In *Clinical Reasoning in the Health Professions*, edited by J. Higgs, S. Loftus, and N. Christensens. Oxford: Butterworth-Heinemann.

HealthEd. 2022. *Your Baby's Funeral*. HE2319. Wellington, NZ: Ministry of Health Manatū Hauora.

Healy, David. 2006. The latest mania: Selling bipolar disorder. *PLoS Medicine* 3 (4):e185.

Henwood, Flis, Sally Wyatt, Angie Hart, and Julie Smith. 2003. "Ignorance is bliss sometimes": Constraints on the emergence of the "informed patient" in the changing landscapes of health information. *Sociology of Health and Illness* 25 (6):589–607.

Heritage, John, and Douglas W. Maynard. 2006. Problems and prospects in the study of physician-patient interaction: 30 years of research. *Annual Review of Sociology* 32 (1):351–74. https://doi.org/10.1146/annurev.soc.32.082905.093959.

Herrick, S. S. 1889. *A Reference Handbook of the Medical Sciences*. Edited by A. H. Buck. Edinburgh: Pentland.

Hesse, Bradford W., David E. Nelson, Gary L. Kreps, Robert T. Croyle, Neeraj K. Arora, Barbara K. Rimer, and Kasisomayajula Viswanath. 2005. Trust and sources of health information: The impact of the internet and its implications for health care providers; findings from the first Health Information National Trends Survey. *Archives of Internal Medicine* 165 (22):2618–24.

Hippocrates. 1983. Prognosis. In *Hippocratic Writings*, edited by G. E. R. Lloyd. London: Penguin.

Hollick, Frederick. 1902. *The Origin of Life and Process of Reproduction in Plants and Animals, With the Anatomy and Physiology of the Human Generative System, Male and Female, and the Causes, Prevention and Cure of the Special Diseases to Which It Is Liable: A Plain, Practical Treatise, for Popular Use*. Philadelphia: David McKay.

Horwitz, Allan V. 2007. Distinguishing distress from disorder as psychological outcomes of stressful social arrangements. *Health* (London) 11 (3):273–89.

Horwitz, Allan V., and Jerome C. Wakefield. 2007. *The Loss of Sadness: How Psychiatry Transformed Normal Sorrow into Depressive Disorder*. New York: Oxford University Press.

Houlihan, Catherine F., Sanjay Patel, David. A. Price, Manoj Valappil, and Uli Schwab. 2010. Life threatening infections labelled swine flu. *British Medical Journal* 340:c137.

Hunt, L. M., E. A. Arndt, H. S. Bell, and H. A. Howard. 2021. Are corporations redefining illness and health? The diabetes epidemic, goal numbers, and blockbuster drugs. *Journal of Bioethical Inquiry* 18:477–497.

Hunter, Kathryn Montgomery. 1991. *Doctors' Stories: The Narrative Structure of Medical Knowledge*. Princeton, NJ: Princeton University Press.

Hydén, Lars-Christer, and Lisbeth Sachs. 1998. Suffering, hope and diagnosis: On the negotiation of chronic fatigue syndrome. *Health* (London) 2 (2):175–93.

Illich, Ivan. 1976. *Limits to Medicine—Medical Nemesis: The Expropriation of Health*. Middlesex, UK: Penguin.

Jackson, Mark. 1996. "Something more than blood": Conflicting accounts of pregnancy loss in eighteenth-century England. In *The Anthropology of Pregnancy Loss: Comparative Studies in Miscarriage, Stillbirth and Neonatal Death*, edited by R. Cecil. Oxford: Berg.

Jackson, Stanley W. 1978. Melancholia and the waning of the humoral theory. *Journal of the History of Medicine and Allied Sciences* 33 (3):367–76.

Jacob, Elin K. 1992. Classification and categorization: Drawing the line. *Advances in Classification Research: Proceedings of the ASIS SIG/DR Classification Research Workshop* 2:67–83.

Jagose, Annamarie. 2003. Against love. Paper delivered to the Department of Cinema Studies, New York University, New York, NY, February 7.

Jaspers, L., F. Feys, W. M. Bramer, O. H. Franco, P. Leusink, and E. M. Laan. 2016. Efficacy and safety of flibanserin for the treatment of hypoactive sexual desire disorder in women: A systematic review and meta-analysis. *JAMA Internal Medicine* 176:453–462.

Jepson, Ruth. 2006. Informed refusal. *Virtual Mentor* 8 (1):24–29.

Jerome, Jerome K. 1889. *Three Men in a Boat (to Say Nothing of the Dog)*. London: J. W. Arrowsmith.

Joffe, Hylton V. August 2015. Summary review for regulatory action. Application number 022526Orig1s000. http://www.accessdata.fda.gov/drugsatfda_docs/nda/2015/022526Orig1s000SumRedt.pdf.

Joinson, Carla. 1992. Coping with compassion fatigue. *Nursing* 22 (4):116, 118–19, 120.

Judicial Watch. 2009. Illegal aliens spread swine flu in US. http://www.judicialwatch.org/blog/2009/04/illegal-aliens-spread-swine-flu-u-s/. Accessed July 28, 2013.

Jutel, Annemarie. 2001. Does size really matter? Weight and values in public health. *Perspectives in Biology and Medicine* 44 (2):283–296.

Jutel, Annemarie. 2005. Weighing health: The moral burden of obesity. *Social Semiotics* 15 (2):113–125.

Jutel, Annemarie. 2006. What's in a name? Death before birth. *Perspectives in Biology and Medicine* 49 (3):425–34.

Jutel, Annemarie. 2008. Doctor's orders: Diagnosis, medicalisation and the exploitation of anti-fat stigma. In *Biopolitics and the "Obesity Epidemic": Governing Bodies*, edited by J. Wright and V. Harwood. New York: Taylor & Francis.

Jutel, Annemarie. 2010a. Framing disease: The example of female hypoactive sexual desire disorder. *Social Science and Medicine* 70:1084–90. https://doi.org/10.1016/j.socscimed.2009.11.040.

Jutel, Annemarie. 2010b. Medically unexplained symptoms and the disease label. *Social Theory and Health* 8:229–45.

Jutel, A. 2013. When pigs could fly: Influenza and the elusive nature of diagnosis. *Perspectives in Biology and Medicine* 56 (4):513–29. https://doi.org/10.1353/pbm.2013.0033.

Jutel, Annemarie. 2016. Truth and lies: Disclosure and the power of diagnosis. *Social Science and Medicine* 165:92–98. https://doi.org/10.1016/j.socscimed.2016.07.037.

Jutel, Annemarie. 2021. Uncertainty and the inconvenient facts of diagnosis. *Endeavour* 45:1–9.

Jutel, Annemarie. 2023. "Between the spaces: Graphic diagnosis." *Perspectives in Biology and Medicine* 66 (2):299–311.

Jutel, Annemarie, and Stephen A. Buetow. 2007. A picture of health? Unmasking the role of appearance in health. *Perspectives in Biology and Medicine* 50 (3):421–34.

Jutel, Annemarie, and Barbara Mintzes. 2017. Female sexual dysfunction: Medicalizing desire. In *Routledge International Handbook of Critical Mental Health*, edited by Bruce M. Z. Cohen, 162–68. Routledge.

Kahn, Eugen. 1957. The life and work of Emil Kraepelin. *Association of Schools of Public Health* 72 (7):527–74.

Kaplan, Helen S. 1977. Hypoactive sexual desire. *Journal of Sex and Marital Therapy* 3 (1):3–9.

Kastelein, J. J., F. Akdim, E. S. Stroes, A. H. Zwinderman, M. L. Bots, A. F. Stalenhoef, F. L. Visseren, E. J. Sijbrands, M. D. Trip, E. A. Stein, et al. 2008. Simvastatin with or without ezetimibe in familial hypercholesterolemia. *New England Journal of Medicine* 358 (14):1431–43.

Kerr, Anne, and Sarah Cunningham-Burley. 2000. On ambivalence and risk: Reflexive modernity and the new human genetics. *Sociology* 34 (2):283–304.

Kilbourne, Jean. 2003. Advertising and disconnection. In *Sex in Advertising*, edited by T. Reichert and J. Lambiase. Mahwah, NJ: Lawrence Erlbaum Associates.

Kipen, H. M., and N. Fiedler. 2002. Environmental factors in medically unexplained symptoms and related syndromes: The evidence and the challenge. *Environmental Health Perspectives* 110 (Suppl. 4):597–99.

Kirmayer, Laurence J., Danielle Groleau, Karl J. Looper, and Melissa D. Dao. 2004. Explaining medically unexplained symptoms. *Canadian Journal of Psychiatry* 49 (10):663–71.

Klawiter, Maren. 1999. Racing for the cure, walking women, and toxic touring: Mapping cultures of action within the Bay Area terrain of breast cancer. *Social Problems* 46 (1):104–26.

Klawiter, Maren. 2008. Moving from Settled to Contested: Transformations in the anatomo-politics of breast cancer, 1970–1990. In *Contesting Illness: Processes and Practice*, edited by Moss Pamela and Teghtsoonian Katherine. Toronto: University of Toronto Press.

Kleinman, Arthur 1988. *The Illness Narratives: Suffering, Healing, and the Human Condition*. New York: Basic Books.

Kleinman, Arthur, Leon Eisenberg, and Byron Good. 1978. Culture, illness, and care: Clinical lessons from anthropologic and cross-cultural research. *Annals of Internal Medicine* 88 (2):251–58.

Klinkenborg, Verlyn. 1994. Dangerous diagnoses. *New Yorker*, July 18:78–80.

Kolker, Emily S. 2004. Framing as a cultural resource in health social movements: Funding activism and the breast cancer movement in the U.S., 1990–1993. *Sociology of Health and Illness* 26 (6):820–44.

Krecke, Albert. 1934. *The doctor and his patients*. London: Kegan Paul, Trench, Trubner.

Kuczmarski, Robert J., and Katherine M. Flegal. 2000. Criteria for definition of overweight in transition: Background and recommendations for the United States. *American Journal of Clinical Nutrition* 72 (5):1074–81.

Kutchins, Herb, and Stuart A. Kirk. 1989. *DSM-III-R*: The conflict over new psychiatric diagnoses. *Health and Social Work* 14 (2):91–101.

Kutchins, Herb, and Stuart A. Kirk. 1997. *Making Us Crazy: "DSM"; The Psychiatric Bible and the Creation of Mental Disorders*. New York: Free Press.

Lacey, C., M. P. Kelly, and A. Jutel. 2020. Fighting words in the antipodes. *Perspectives in Biology and Medicine* 63 (4): 669–82. https://doi.org/10.1353/pbm.2020.0054.

Laking, George, Joanne Lord, and Alastair Fischer. 2006. The economics of diagnosis. *Health Economics* 15 (10):1109–20.

Lancet. 1897. Notes, short comments and answers to correspondents: The reliance personal weighing machine. May 8:1316.

Lancet. 1899. New inventions. April 2:940.

Lapham, Roger. F. 1937. *Disease and the Man.* Oxford: Oxford University Press.

Laqueur, Thomas. 1990. *Making Sex: Body and Gender from the Greeks to Freud.* Cambridge, MA: Harvard University Press.

Lavater, John Caspar. 1855. *Essays on Physiognomy—Designed to Promote Knowledge and Harmony among Mankind.* 15th ed. Translated by T. Holcroft. London: William Tegg.

Lawn, J. E., M. Y. Yakoob, R. A. Haws, T. Soomro, G. L. Darmstadt, and Z. A. Bhutta. 2009. 3.2 million stillbirths: Epidemiology and overview of the evidence review. *BMC Pregnancy Childbirth* 9 (Suppl. 1):S2.

Leder, Drew. 1990. Clinical interpretation: The hermeneutics of medicine. *Theoretical Medicine* 11:9–24.

Lee, Jennifer A., and Cat J. Pause. 2016. Stigma in practice: Barriers to health for fat women. *Frontiers in Psychology* 7:1–15. https://doi.org/10.3389/fpsyg.2016.02063.

Lee, R. 2021. B.1.1.7: What we know about the novel SARS-CoV-2 variant; What is the new SARS-CoV-2 variant and why is it important? *American Society for Microbiology.* https://asm.org/Articles/2021/January/B-1-1-7-What-We-Know-About-the-Novel-SARS-CoV-2-Va.

Lee, Shirley, and Avis Mysyk. 2004. The medicalization of compulsive buying. *Social Science and Medicine* 58 (9):1709–18.

Lemon, George William. 1701. *English Etymology; or a Derivative Dictionary of the English Language in Two Alphabets.* London: G. Robinson.

Leray, Jean. 1931. *Embonpoint et obésité: Conceptions et thérapeutiques actuelles.* Paris: Massion et Cie.

Levine, Hallie. 2022. Do I have long COVID? Here's how to tell. *WebMD.* https://www.webmd.com/covid/news/20220719/do-i-have-long-covid. Accessed August 3, 2022.

Lexchin, Joel. 2006. Bigger and better: How Pfizer redefined erectile dysfunction. *PLoS Medicine* 3 (4):1–4.

Lief, Harold I. 1977. Inhibited sexual desire. *Medical Aspects of Human Sexuality* 7:94–95.

Light, Donald, and Sol Levine. 1988. The changing character of the medical profession: A theoretical overview. *Milbank Quarterly* 66:10–32.

Lippman, Abby. 1991. Prenatal genetic testing and screening: Constructing needs and reinforcing inequities. *American Journal of Law and Medicine* 17 (1/2):15–50.

Locker, David. 1981. *Symptoms and Illness: The Cognitive Organization of Disorder.* London: Tavistock.

Lombroso, Caesar, and William Ferrero. 1895. *The Female Offender.* London: T. Fisher Unwin.

Lorber, J. 1997. *Gender and the Social Construction of Illness.* Thousand Oaks, CA: Sage.

Lorber, Judith, and Lisa Jean Moore. 2002. *Gender and the Social Construction of Illness.* Walnut Creek, CA: Alta Mira Press.

Lunbeck, Elizabeth. 1987. "A new generation of women": Progressive psychiatrists and the hypersexual female. *Feminist Studies* 13 (3):513–43.

Lupton, Deborah, and Annemarie Jutel. 2015. "It's like having a physician in your pocket!": A critical analysis of self-diagnosis smartphone apps. *Social Science and Medicine* 133:128–35.

Mahajan, A. P., J. N. Sayles, V. A. Patel, R. H. Remien, S. R. Sawires, D. J. ORTIZ, G. Szekeres, and T. J. Coates. 2008. Stigma in the HIV/AIDS epidemic: A review of the literature and recommendations for the way forward. *AIDS* (London) 22 (suppl. 2): S67–S79.

Malterud, Kirsti. 1999. The (gendered) construction of diagnosis interpretation of medical signs in women patients. *Theoretical Medicine and Bioethics* 20 (3):275–86.

Malterud, Kirsti. 2000. Symptoms as a source of medical knowledge: Understanding medically unexplained disorders in women. *Family Medicine* 32 (9):603–11.

Malterud, Kirsti. 2001. Subjective symptoms without objective findings: A challenge for theory and practice of general medicine. *Ugeskr Laeger* 163 (48):6729–34.

Malterud, Kirsti. 2005. Humiliation instead of care? *Lancet* 9488:785–86.

Malterud, Kirsti, Lucy Candid, and Lorraine Code. 2004. Responsible and responsive knowing in medical diagnosis: The medical gaze revisited. *NORA: Nordic Journal of Feminist and Gender Research* 12 (1):8–19.

Malterud, Kirsti, and A. Taksdal. 2007. Shared spaces of reflection: Approaching the medically unexplained disorder. *Junctures: The Journal for Thematic Dialogue* (9):27–38.

Mamo, L., and J. R. Fosket. 2009. Scripting the body: Pharmaceuticals and the (re) making of menstruation. *Signs: Journal of Women in Culture and Society* 34:925–49.

Marcus, Pamela M., Eric J. Bergstralh, Mark H. Zweig, Ann Harris, Kenneth P. Offord, and Robert S. Fontana. 2006. Extended lung cancer incidence follow-up in the Mayo Lung Project and overdiagnosis. *Journal of the National Cancer Institute* 98 (11):748–56.

Mayes, Rick, and Allen V. Horwitz. 2005. *DSM-III* and the revolution in the classification of mental illness. *Journal of the History of the Behavioral Sciences* 41 (3):249–67.

McEntee, Michael. 2003. Health screenings: A tool for today's marketers. *Medical Marketing and Media* 38 (2):52–59.

McEwan, Ian. 2004. The diagnosis. *New Yorker,* December 20:116–29.

McKay, B. 2020. Virus in China is part of a growing threat: New type of so-called coronavirus is possible cause of the outbreak in the city of Wuhan. *Wall Street Journal,* January 10.

McKinlay, Eileen. 2005. Men and health: A literature review. Wellington, NZ: Department of General Practice, Wellington School of Medicine and Health Sciences, Otago.

McLeod, C., A. Bagust, A. Boland, P. Dagenais, R. Dickson, Y. Dundar, R. A. Hill,

A. Jones, R. Mujica Mota, and T. Walley. 2007. Adalimumab, etanercept and in-fliximab for the treatment of ankylosing spondylitis: A systematic review and eco-nomic evaluation. *Health Technology Assessment* 11 (28):iii–iv, 1–158.

Meador, Clifton. 2005. *Symptoms of Unknown Origin: A Medical Odyssey.* Nashville: Vanderbilt University Press.

Melechi, Antonio. 2003. *Fugitive Minds: On Madness, Sleep and Other Twilight Afflic-tions.* London: Arrow Books.

Melendy, Mary Ries. 1904. *Vivilore: The Pathway to Mental and Physical Perfection.* Wellington, NZ: Milton Porter.

Mendelson, George. 2003. Homosexuality and psychiatric nosology. *Australian and New Zealand Journal of Psychiatry* 37 (6):678–83.

Meyer-Kleinmann, Julia. 2008a. Largest study of its kind reveals low sexual desire is most common female sexual problem. *Boehringer Ingelheim Science and Technology Communications,* October 31.

Meyer-Kleinmann, Julia. 2008b. Women suffering from decreased sexual desire: Si-lence hinders diagnosis of the prevalent condition hypoactive sexual desire disorder (HSDD). *Boehringer Ingelheim Science and Technology Communications,* May 7.

Miller, F. 2006. Redefining disease? The nosologic implications of molecular genetic knowledge. *Perspectives in Biology and Medicine* 49 (1):99–114.

Miller, Fiona A., Megan E. Begbie, Mita Giacomini, Catherine Ahern, and Erin A. Harvey. 2006. Redefining disease? The nosologic implications of molecular ge-netic knowledge. *Perspectives in Biology and Medicine* 49 (1):99–114.

Miller, Genevieve. 1962. "Airs, waters, and places" in history. *Journal of the History of Medicine and Allied Sciences* 17 (1):129–40.

Milliken, Donald. 1998. Death by restraint. *Canadian Medical Association Journal* 158 (12):1611–12.

Mills, Wilfred. 1977. Definition of perinatal mortality. *Lancet,* June 25:1358.

Mintzes, Barbara, Morris L. Barer, Richard L. Kravitz, Arminee Kazanjian, Ken Bas-sett, Joel Lexchin, Robert G. Evans, Richard Pan, and Stephen A. Marion. 2002. Influence of direct to consumer pharmaceutical advertising and patients' requests on prescribing decisions: Two site cross sectional survey. *British Medical Journal* 324 (7332):278–79.

Mirowsky, John, and Catherine E. Ross. 1989. Psychiatric diagnosis as reified mea-surement. *Journal of Health and Social Behavior* 30 (1):11–25, discussion on 26–40.

Moncrieff, Joanna, Steve Hopker, and Philip Thomas. 2005. Psychiatry and the phar-maceutical industry: Who pays the piper? *Psychiatric Bulletin* 29:84–85.

Monistat. 2023. We've all been there. Doctor discussion guide. https://www.monistat.com/sites/monistat/files/2019-12/Doctor%20Discussion%20Guide.pdf. Accessed June 6, 2023.

Morse, Janice M. 2006. The politics of evidence. *Qualitative Health Research* 16 (3):395–404.

Moynihan, Ray. 2003. The making of a disease: Female sexual dysfunction. *British Medical Journal* 326 (7379):45–47.

Moynihan, Ray, and Alan Cassels. 2005. *Selling Sickness: How Drug Companies Are Turning Us All into Patients.* Sydney: Allen & Unwin.

Moynihan, Ray, Iona Heath, and David Henry. 2002. Selling sickness: The pharmaceutical industry and disease mongering. *British Medical Journal* 324 (7342):886–91.

Mullen, Patricia D. 1997. Compliance becomes concordance. *British Medical Journal* 314 (7082):691–92.

Munro, Robin J. 2002. Political psychiatry in post-Mao China and its origins in the cultural revolution. *Journal of the American Academy of Psychiatry and the Law* 30 (1):97–106.

Murray, T. Jock. 2005. *Multiple Sclerosis: The History of a Disease.* New York: Demos Medical.

Napheys, George H. 1871. *The Physical Life of Woman: Advice to the Maiden, Wife and Mother* 6th ed. Philadelphia: George Maclean.

Nerlich, B., and C. Halliday. 2007. Avian flu: The creation of expectations in the interplay between science and the media. *Sociology of Health and Illness* 29:46–65.

Nettleton, Sarah. 2004. The emergence of e-scaped medicine. *Sociology* 38 (4):661–79.

Nettleton, Sarah. 2006. "I just want permission to be ill": Towards a sociology of medically unexplained symptoms. *Social Science and Medicine* 62 (5):1167–78.

Nettleton, Sarah, Lisa O'Malley, Ian Watt, and Philip Duffey. 2004. Enigmatic illness: Narratives of patients who live with medically unexplained symptoms. *Social Theory and Health* 2:47–66.

Neuberger, Julia. 1999. Do we need a new word for patients? Let's do away with "patients." *British Medical Journal* 318:1756–57.

Nevill, Alan M., Arthur D. Stewart, Tim Olds, and Roger Holder. 2006. Relationship between adiposity and body size reveals limitations of BMI. *American Journal of Physical Anthropology* 129:151–56.

New Zealand College of Midwives. 2018. *Midwifery Standards Review Handbook.* Christchurch, NZ: New Zealand College of Midwives.

New Zealand Government. 2020. *Unite against COVID-19.* https://covid19.govt.nz/. Accessed October 2, 2020.

Nilsson, P. M., J. A. Nilsson, B. Hedblad, G. Berglund, and F. Lindgarde. 2002. The enigma of increased non-cancer mortality after weight loss in healthy men who are overweight or obese. *Journal of Internal Medicine* 252 (1):70–78.

Novak, Michael. 1965. Toward understanding Aristotle's categories. *Philosophy and Phenomenological Research* 26 (1):117–23.

Novo Nordisk. 2023. Find the tools you need to move forward. https://www.saxenda.com/support-and-resources/tools-and-resources.html. Accessed August 3, 2023.

NZ Parliamentary Counsel Office. 1961. Crimes Act, section 181, "Concealing the dead body of child." https://www.legislation.govt.nz/act/public/1961/0043/latest/DLM329350.html?search=sw_096be8ed81d369a9_warrantless_25_se&p=1&tagf=1.

Ockham, William of. 1997. In *Chambers Biographical Dictionary*, edited by M. Parry. New York: Chambers.

Oliver, J. Eric. 2006. The politics of pathology: How obesity became an epidemic disease. *Perspectives in Biology and Medicine* 49 (4):611–29.

One News. 2005. Baby Aaron's mother found. March 9. https://www.nzherald.co .nz/hawkes-bay-today/news/top-story-baby-aarons-mum-found/P76XSCXDWSE 6NCCLDTKUH2XCNI/.

Oran, D. P., and E. J. Topol. 2020. Prevalence of asymptomatic SARS-CoV-2 infection. *Annals of Internal Medicine* 173:362–67.

Orpana, Heather M., Jean-Mari Berthelot, Mark S. Kaplan, David H. Feeny, Bentson McFarland, and Nancy A. Ross. 2009. BMI and mortality: Results from a national longitudinal study of Canadian adults. *Obesity* 18 (1): 214–18.

Ovid. 1985. *Metamorphoses*. Book 3. Translated and edited by D. E. Hill. Warminster, UK: Aris & Phillips.

Pabst Brewing. 1897. Pabst Malt Extract. *Godey's*, January, 115.

Packard, R. M., P. J. Brown, R. L. Berkelman, and H. Frumkin (Eds.). 2004. *Emerging Illnesses and Society: Negotiating the Public Health Agenda*. Baltimore: Johns Hopkins University Press.

Paquette, Mary. 2003. Excited delirium: Does it exist? *Perspectives in Psychiatric Care* 39 (3):93–94.

Parry, Vince. 2007. Disease branding: What is it, why it works, and how to do it. *Pharmaceutical Executive*, October:22–24.

Parsons, Talcott. 1951. Illness and the role of the physician: A sociological perspective. *American Journal of Orthopsychiatry* 21:452–60.

Parsons, Talcott. 1958. Definitions of health and illness in the light of American values and social structure. In *Patients, Physicians and Illness: Sourcebook in Behavioral Science and Medicine*, edited by E. G. Jaco. Glencoe, IL: Free Press.

Payer, Lynn. 1992. *Disease-Mongers: How Doctors, Drug Companies, and Insurers Are Making You Feel Sick*. New York: John Wiley & Sons.

Percival, Thomas. 1985. *Medical Ethics; Or, A Code of Institutes and Precepts, Adapted to the Professional Conduct of Physicians and Surgeons*. Birmingham, AL: Classics of Medicine Library.

Petchesky, Rosalind P. 1987. Fetal images: The power of visual culture in the politics of reproduction. *Feminist Studies* 13 (2):263–92.

Petersen, Alan, and Karen Pienarr. 2024. Competing realities, uncertain diagnoses of infectious disease: Mass self-testing for COVID-19 and liminal bio-citizenship. *Sociology of Health and Illness* [full publication details forthcoming].

Petites études de la nature ou entretiens recréatifs d'une mère avec ses deux filles sur l'histoire naturelle des animaux et des plantes: Les phénomenes astronomiques, et les progrès des arts, des sciences et de la civilisation. 1840. Paris: Niogret.

Pharmac. 2023. Application for subsidy by special authority. https://schedule.pharmac .govt.nz/2023/12/01/SA2178.pdf. Accessed December 15, 2023.

Pilowsky, Issy. 1994. Abnormal illness behaviour: A 25th anniversary review. *Australia New Zealand Journal of Psychiatry* 28:566–73.

Pratt, Lois, Arthur Seligmann, and George Reader. 1958. Physicians' views on the level of medical information among patients. In *Patients, Physicians and Illness: Sourcebook in Behavioral Science and Medicine*, edited by E. G. Jaco. Glencoe, IL: Free Press.

Prause, Nicole, and Cynthia A. Graham. 2007. Asexuality: classification and characterization. *Archives of Sexual Behavior* 36 (3):341–56.

Procter & Gamble. 2009. Beautify your heart. www.metamucil.com/beautify-your-heart/resources-bmi-calculator.php (site discontinued). Accessed September 30, 2009.

Proctor, S. P., T. Heeren, R. F. White, J. Wolfe, M. S. Borgos, J. D. Davis, L. Pepper, R. Clapp, P. B. Sutker, J. J. Vasterling, and D. Ozonoff. 1998. Health status of Persian Gulf War veterans: Self-reported symptoms, environmental exposures and the effect of stress. *International Journal of Epidemiology* 27 (6):1000–1010.

Puhl, Rebecca. M., and Kelly D. Brownell. 2003. Psychosocial origins of obesity stigma: Toward changing a powerful and pervasive bias. *Obesity Reviews* 4:213–27.

Puhl, Rebecca M., and Chelsea A. Heuer. 2009. The stigma of obesity: A review and update. *Obesity* 17 (5):941–64. https://doi.org/10.1038/oby.2008.636.

Quetelet, Adolphe. 1870. *Anthropométrie, ou, Mesure des différentes facultés de l'homme.* Paris: C. Muquardt.

Raz, Aviad E. 2009. Eugenic utopias/dystopias, reprogenetics, and community genetics. *Sociology of Health and Illness* 31 (4):602–16.

Raz, Aviad E., and Yafa Vizner. 2009. Carrier matching and collective socialization in community genetics: Dor Yeshorim and the reinforcement of stigma. *Social Science and Medicine* 67 (9):1361–69.

Reagan, Leslie. J. 2003. From hazard to blessing to tragedy: Representations of miscarriage in twentieth-century America. *Feminist Studies* 13 (2):263–92.

Rebbeck, Timothy R., Tara Friebel, Henry T. Lynch, Susan L. Neuhausen, Laura van't Veer, Judy E. Garber, Gareth R. Evans, Steven A. Narod, Claudine Isaacs, Ellen Matloff, et al. 2004. Bilateral prophylactic mastectomy reduces breast cancer risk in BRCA1 and BRCA2 mutation carriers: The PROSE Study Group. *Journal of Clinical Oncology* 22 (6):1055–62.

Rector, Frank L. 1936. Seven steps to the undertaker. *Bulletin of the American Society for the Control of Cancer*:181–85.

Reichert, Tom, and Jacqueline Lambiase. 2003. One phenomenon, multiple lenses: Bridging perspectives to examine sex in advertising. In *Sex in Advertising: Perspectives on the Erotic Appeal*, edited by T. Reichert and J. Lambiase. Mahwah, NJ: Lawrence Erlbaum Associates.

Reventlow, Susanne D., Lotte Hvas, and Kirsti Malterud. 2006. Making the invisible body visible: Bone scans, osteoporosis and women's bodily experiences. *Social Science and Medicine* 62 (11):2720–31.

Revista de enfermeria. 1989. La fatiga de la compasión. Editorial. 12 (136):9.

Rhodes, Lorna A., Carol A. McPhillips-Tangum, Christine Markham, and Rebecca

Klenk. 1999. The power of the visible: The meaning of diagnostic tests in chronic back pain. *Social Science and Medicine* 48 (9):1189–203.

Richardson, Diane. 2007. Patterned fluidities: (Re)imagining the relationship between gender and sexuality. *Sociology* 41 (3):457–74.

Richardson, Ernest Cushing. 1901. *Classification*. New York: Charles Scribner's sons.

Roberts, Mary Louise. 1998. Gender, Consumption, and Commodity Culture. *American Historical Review* 103 (3):817–44.

Robins, Lee N., and John E. Helzer. 1986. Diagnosis and clinical assessment: The current state of psychiatric diagnosis. *Annual Review of Psychology* 37:409–32.

Robinson, G. Canby. 1939. *The Patient as Person: A Study of the Social Aspects of Illness*. New York: Commonwealth Fund.

Robinson, K., P. F. Whelan, O. Ghita, and D. Brennan. 2005. Measurement and localization of body fat in whole body MRI. Third Annual IEI Biomedical Engineering Research Award, Dublin.

Rodin, Mari. 1992. The social construction of premenstrual syndrome. *Social Science and Medicine* 35 (1):49–56.

Rogler, Lloyd H. 1997. Making sense of historical changes in the *Diagnostic and Statistical Manual of Mental Disorders*: Five propositions. *Journal of Health and Social Behavior* 38 (1):9–20.

Romero-Corral, Abel, Victor M. Montori, Virend K. Somers, Josef Korinek, Randal J. Thomas, Thomas G. Allison, Farouk Mookadam, and Francisco Lopez-Jimenez. 2006. Association of bodyweight with total mortality and with cardiovascular events in coronary artery disease: A systematic review of cohort studies. *Lancet* (368):666–78.

Rosecrance, John. 1985. Compulsive gambling and the medicalization of deviance. *Social Problems* 32 (3):275–84.

Rosenberg, Charles E. 1992. *Explaining Epidemics and Other Studies in the History of Medicine*. Cambridge: Cambridge University Press.

Rosenberg, Charles E. 2002. The tyranny of diagnosis: Specific entities and individual experience. *Milbank Quarterly* 80 (2):237–60.

Rosenberg, Charles E. 2006. Contested boundaries: Psychiatry, disease, and diagnosis. *Perspectives in Biology and Medicine* 49 (3):407–24.

Rosenberg, Charles E., and Janet Golden (Eds.). 1992. *Framing Disease: Studies in Cultural History*. New Brunswick, NJ: Rutgers University Press.

Rothblum, Esther D., and Kathleen A. Brehony. 1993. *Boston Marriages: Romantic but Asexual Relationships among Contemporary Lesbians*. Amherst: University of Massachusetts Press.

Rothwell, David J. 1985. Requirements of a national health information system. In *Role of Informatics in Health Data Coding and Classification Systems*, edited by R. A. Cole, D. J. Protti, and J. R. Scherrer. Amsterdam: Elsevier.

Rowley, M. J., M. J. Hensley, M. W. Brinsmead, and J. H. Wlodarczyk. 1995. Continuity of care by a midwife team versus routine care during pregnancy and birth: A randomised trial. *Medical Journal of Australia* 163 (6):289–93.

Ryall, Tony. 2007. Prostate cancer guidelines taking too long. New Zealand National Party press release. www.scoop.co.nz/stories/PA0701/S00063.htm.

Sabo, Brenda M. 2006. Compassion fatigue and nursing work: Can we accurately capture the consequences of caring work? *International Journal of Nursing Practice* 12 (3):136–42.

Sarbin, Theodore R., and John I. Kitsuse. 1994. *Constructing the Social: Inquiries in Social Construction*. London: Sage.

Scambler, G. 2009. Health-related stigma. *Sociology of Health and Illness* 31:441–55.

Scherrer, Kristin S. 2008. Coming to an asexual identity: Negotiating identity, negotiating desire. *Sexualities* 11 (5):621–41.

Schrader, Catharina. 1987. *"Mother and Child Were Saved": The Memoirs (1693–1740) of the Frisian Midwife Catharina Schrader*. Translated by H. Marland. Amsterdam: Editions Rodophi.

Schwartz, Hillel. 1986. *Never Satisfied: A Cultural History of Diets, Fantasies, and Fat.* New York: Anchor Books.

Schwartz, Lisa M., Steven Woloshin, Floyd J. Fowler Jr., and H. Giblert Welch. 2004. Enthusiasm for cancer screening in the United States. *Journal of the American Medical Association* 291 (1):71–78.

Scott, Susie. 2006. The medicalisation of shyness: From social misfits to social fitness. *Sociology of Health and Illness* 28 (2):133–53.

Scott, Wilbur, J. 1990. PTSD in *DSM-III*: A case in the politics of diagnosis and disease. *Social Problems* 37 (3):294–310.

Sharpe, M. 2002. Medically unexplained symptoms and syndromes. *Clinical Medicine* 2 (6): 501–4.

al-Shaykh, Hanan. 1994. Inside a Moroccan bath. In *Minding the Body: Women Writers on Body and Soul*, edited by P. Foster. New York: Doubleday.

Sheffield Hearing Voices Network. 2010. Hearing voices network. www.hearing-voices.org. Accessed June 10, 2010.

Shermis, Sherwin S. 1962. What makes a subject respectable? On becoming an intellectual discipline. *Phi Delta Kappan* 44 (2):84–86.

Sherson, Venitia. 2010. Caring till it hurts. *Dominion Post*, 13 March, suppl.:8–11.

Shifren, Jan L., Brigitta U. Monz, Patricia A. Russo, Anthony Segreti, and Catherine B. Johannes. 2008. Sexual problems and distress in United States women: Prevalence and correlates. *Obstetrics and Gynecology* 112 (5):970–78.

Shorter, Edward. 1992. *From Paralysis to Fatigue: A History of Psychosomatic Illness in the Modern Era*. New York: Free Press.

Shutzberg, Mani. 2021. The doctor as parent, partner, provider . . . or comrade? Distribution of power in past and present models of the doctor-patient relationship. *Health Care Analysis* 29:231–48.

Sills, Terrence, Glen Wunderlich, Robert Pyke, R. Taylor Segraves, Sandra Leiblum, Anita Clayton, Dan Cotton, and Kenneth Evans. 2005. The Sexual Interest and Desire Inventory–Female (SIDI-F): Item response analyses of data from women diagnosed with hypoactive sexual desire disorder. *Journal of Sexual Medicine* 2 (6):801–18.

Silvestri, L. G., and L. R. Hill. 1964. Some problems of the taxometric approach. In *Phenetic and Phylogenetic Classification*, edited by V. H. Heywood and J. McNeill. London: Systematics Association.

Sim, Julius, and Sue Madden. 2008. Illness experience in fibromyalgia syndrome: A metasynthesis of qualitative studies. *Social Science and Medicine* 67 (1):57–67.

Skegg, Keren. 1993. Multiple sclerosis presenting as a pure psychiatric disorder. *Psychological Medicine* 23 (4):909–14.

Smith-Rosenberg, C., and C. Rosenberg. 1973. The female animal: Medical and biological views of woman and her role in nineteenth-century America. *Journal of American History* 60 (2):332–56.

Sokal, Robert R. 1974. Classification: Purposes, principles, progress, prospects. *Science* 185 (4157):1115–23.

Solve ME/CFS Initiative. 2023. Do I have ME/CFS? Quiz. https://solvecfs.org/me-cfs-long-covid/do-i-have-mecfs-quiz/. Accessed December 15, 2023.

Sontag, Susan. 1978. *Illness as Metaphor.* New York: Farrar, Straus and Giroux.

Sotgiu, G., and C. C. Dobler. 2020. Social stigma in the time of Coronavirus. *European Respiratory Journal* 56 (2):2002461.

Sotiriou, Christos, Soek-Ying Neo, Lisa M. McShane, Edward L. Korn, Philip M. Long, Amir Jazaeri, Philippe Martiat, Steve B. Fox, Adrian L. Harris, and Edison T. Liu. 2003. Breast cancer classification and prognosis based on gene expression profiles from a population-based study. *Proceedings of the National Academy of Sciences of the United States of America* 100 (18):10393–98.

Spitzack, Carole. 1990. *Confessing Excess: Women and the Politics of Body Reduction.* Albany: State University of New York Press.

Stafford, Barbara, John La Puma, and David Schiedermayer. 1989. One face of beauty, one picture of health: The hidden aesthetic of medical practice. *Journal of Medicine and Philosophy* 14:213–30.

Star, Susan Leigh, and Geoffrey C. Bowker. 1997. Of lungs and lungers: The classified story of tuberculosis. *Mind, Culture, and Activity* 4 (1):3–23.

Star, Susan Leigh, and James R. Griesemer. 1989. Institutional ecology, "translations" and boundary objects: Amateurs and professionals in Berkeley's Museum of Vertebrate Zoology, 1907–39. *Social Studies of Science* 19 (3):387–420.

Stephenson, N., and M. Jamieson. 2009. Securitising health: Australian newspaper coverage of pandemic influenza. *Sociology of Health and Illness* 31:525–39.

Stewart, J. A. 1814. *The Young Woman's Companion; or, Female Instructor: Being a Sure and Complete Guide to Every Acquirement Essential in Forming a Pleasing Companion, a Respectable Mother, or a Useful Member of Society.* Oxford: Bartlett and Newman.

Stewart, Jonathan T. 1989. Misdiagnosis of Huntington's disease. *Journal of Neuropsychiatry and Clinical Neurosciences* 1 (1):97.

Stone, Jon, Wojtek Wojcik, Daniel Durrance, Alan Carson, Steff Lewis, Lesley Mac-

Kenzie, Charles P. Warlow, and Michael Sharpe. 2002. What should we say to patients with symptoms unexplained by disease? The "number needed to offend." *British Medical Journal* 325 (7378):1449–50.

St-Onge, Myreille, Helene Provencher, and Carl Ouellet. 2005. Entendre des voix: Nouvelles voies ouvrant sur la pratique et la recherche. *Sante mentale au Quebec* 30 (1):125–50.

Straussner, S. Lala A. 2013. The *DSM-5* diagnostic criteria: What's new? *Journal of Social Work Practice in the Addictions* 13 (4):448–53. https://doi.org/10.1080/1533256X .2013.840199.

Stuff. 2020. We're all in this together. March 31. https://www.stuff.co.nz/national /health/coronavirus/120670237/covid19-were-all-in-this-together.

Swayne, Jeremy. 1993. A common language of care? *Journal of Interprofessional Care* 7 (1):29–35.

Sydenham, Thomas. 1742. *The entire works of Dr Thomas Sydenham, newly made English from the originals: [. . .] To which are added, explanatory and practical notes, from the best medicinal writers. By John Swan, M.D.* London: printed for Edward Cave.

Sykes, William S. 1927. *A Manual of General Medical Practice.* H. K. Lewis.

Temple, Robert. 1999. Are surrogate markers adequate to assess cardiovascular disease drugs? *Journal of the American Medical Association* 282 (8):790–95.

Thomas, Joseph. 1891. *A Complete Pronouncing Medical Dictionary.* London: Deacon.

Tiefer, Leonore. 1996. The medicalization of sexuality: Conceptual, normative, and professional issues. *Annual Review of Sex Research* 7:252–82.

Tiefer, Leonore. 2006. Female sexual dysfunction: A case study of disease mongering and activist resistance. *PLoS Medicine* 3 (4):e178.

Timmermans, Stefan, and Marc Berg. 2003. The practice of medical technology. *Sociology of Health and Illness* 25 (3):97–114.

Trundle, Catherine. 2010. Commonwealth nuclear test veterans and the quest for recognition. In *Graduate School of Nursing, Midwifery and Health Research Seminar Series.* Victoria, NZ: University of Wellington.

Turner, Richard C. 2007. Theorizing an emerging discipline: Philanthropic studies. *Nonprofit and Voluntary Sector Quarterly* 36 (4, suppl.):163S–68S.

Undeland, Merete, and Kirsti Malterud. 2002. Diagnostic work in general practice: More than naming a disease. *Scandinavian Journal of Primary Health Care* 20 (3):145–50.

Veith, Ilza. 1981. Historical reflections on the changing concepts of disease. In *Concepts of Health and Disease: Interdisciplinary Perspectives,* edited by A. L. Caplan, H. T. Engelhardt Jr., and J. J. McCartney. Reading, MA: Addison-Wesley.

Vertinsky, Patricia A. 1994. *The Eternally Wounded Woman: Women, Doctors, and Exercise in the Late Nineteenth Century.* Urbana: University of Illinois Press.

Wahab, M. A., E. M. Nickless, R. Najar-M'kacher, C. Parmentier, J. V. Podd, and R. E. Rowland. 2008. Elevated chromosome translocation frequencies in New Zealand nuclear test veterans. *Cytogenetic and Genome Research* 121 (2):79–87.

Wailoo, Keith. 1997. *Drawing Blood: Technology and Disease Identity in Twentieth-Century America.* Baltimore: Johns Hopkins University Press.

Waldenstrom, U., and D. Turnbull. 1998. A systematic review comparing continuity of midwifery care with standard maternity services. *British Journal of Obstetrics and Gynaecology* 105 (11):1160–70.

Walzl, Dennis, Andrew J. Solomon, and Jon Stone. 2022. Functional neurological disorder and multiple sclerosis: A systematic review of misdiagnosis and clinical overlap. *Journal of Neurology* 269 (2):654–63. https://doi.org/10.1007/s00415-021-10436-6.

Ware, Norma C. 1992. Social construction of illness: The delegitimation of illness experience in chronic fatigue syndrome. *Medical Anthropology Quarterly* 6 (4):347–61.

Weinberg, Darin. 2021. Diagnosis as topic and as resource: Reflections on the epistemology and ontology of disease in medical sociology. *Symbolic Interaction* 44: 367–391.

Wessley, S. 2002. Medically unexplained symptoms and syndromes. *Clinical Medicine* 2 (6): 501–4.

WHO (World Health Organization). 1957. *Manual of the International Statistical Classification of Diseases, Injuries and Causes of Death.* Geneva: WHO.

WHO (World Health Organization). 1977. *International Statistical Classification of Diseases and Related Health Problems* (9th revision). Geneva: WHO.

WHO (World Health Organization). 1993. *International Statistical Classification of Diseases and Related Health Problems* (10th revision). Geneva: WHO.

WHO (World Health Organization). 2016. *Making Every Baby Count: Audit and Review of Still Births and Neonatal Deaths.* Geneva: World Health Organization.

WHO (World Health Organization). 2020. WHO COVID-19 case definition: 16 December 2020. *COVID-19: Surveillance, case investigation and epidemiological protocols.* https://www.who.int/publications/i/item/WHO-2019-nCoV-Surveillance_Case _Definition-2020.2 (site discontinued). Accessed March 7, 2021.

WHO (World Health Organization). 2021. Influenza at the human-animal interface: Summary and assessment, from 16 April to 21 May 2021. https://cdn.who.int/media /docs/default-source/influenza/human-animal-interface-risk-assessments/influenza _summary_ira_ha_interface_may_2021.pdf?sfvrsn=d75e4b5c_7&download=true. Accessed December 14, 2023.

WHO (World Health Organization). 2023a. Controlling the obesity epidemic. https:// www.who.int/activities/controlling-the-global-obesity-epidemic. Accessed November 28, 2023.

WHO (World Health Organization). 2023b. WHO Family of International Classification (FIC). https://www.who.int/standards/classifications. Accessed November 28, 2023.

Whooley, Owen. 2017. DSM and the spectre of ignorance: Psychiatric classification as a tool of professional power. In *Routledge International Handbook of Critical Mental Health,* edited by Bruce M. Z. Cohen, 179–185. New York: Routledge.

Whooley, Owen. 2019. *On the Heels of Ignorance: Psychiatry and the Politics of Not Knowing.* Chicago: University of Chicago Press.

Whooley, O., and A. V. Horwitz. 2013. The paradox of professional success: Grand ambition, furious resistance, and the derailment of the *DSM-5* revision process. In

Making the DSM-5: Concepts and Controversies, edited by J. Paris and J. Phillips, 75–92. New York: Springer. https://doi.org/10.1007/978-1-4614-6504-1_6.

Williamson, Charlotte. 1999. The challenge of lay partnership: It provides a different view of the world. *British Medical Journal* 319 (7212):721–22.

Willis, Thomas. 1681. *The Remaining Medical Works of that Famous and Renowned Physician Dr Thomas Willis*. London: T. Dring, C. Harper, J. Leigh, and S. Martyn.

Wilson, Patricia M. 2001. A policy analysis of the expert patient in the United Kingdom: Self-care as an expression of pastoral power? *Health and Social Care in the Community* 9 (3):134–42.

Winkelman, Warren J., and Chun Wei Choo. 2003. Provider-sponsored virtual communities for chronic patients: Improving health outcomes through organizational patient-centered knowledge management. *Health Expectations* 6 (4):352–58.

Wolfe, David E. 1961. Sydenham and Locke on the limits of anatomy. *Bulletin of the History of Medicine* 35:193–220.

Wolinsky, Howard. 2005. Disease mongering and drug marketing. *European Molecular Biology Organization Reports* 6 (7):612–14.

Woloshin, Steven., and Lisa M. Schwartz. 2016. US Food and Drug Administration approval of Flibanserin: Even the score does not add up. *JAMA Internal Medicine* 176:439–42.

Wolters, R., C. Wensing, C. Van Weel, G. J. Van der Wilt, and R. P. T. M. Grol. 2002. Lower urinary tract symptoms: Social influence is more important than symptoms in seeking medical care. *British Journal of Urology International* 90:655–61.

Women's Health Committee. 2021. *Maternal and Perinatal Data Collection*. Victoria, AU: Royal Australia New Zealand College of Obstetricians and Gynaecologists.

Wooldridge, F. 2009. Swine flu-immigration, death and disease . . . and consequences for Americas. *Alt News*. http://rense.com/general85/sw.htm. Accessed 28 July 2013.

World Obesity. 2023. Global obesity observatory: Cook Islands. https://data.world obesity.org/country/cook-islands-46/. Accessed December 15, 2023.

Yip, Kam-Shing. 2005. An historical review of the mental health services in the People's Republic of China. *International Journal of Social Psychiatry* 51 (2):106–18.

Yudkin, J. S., and V. M. Montori. 2014. The epidemic of pre-diabetes: The medicine and the politics. *British Medical Journal* 349:4485.

Zavestoski, Stephen, Phil Brown, Meadow Linder, Sabrina McCormick, and Brian Mayer. 2002. Science, policy, activism, and war: Defining the health of Gulf War veterans. *Science, Technology, and Human Values* 27 (2):171–205.

Zerubavel, Eviatar. 1991. *The Fine Line: Making Distinctions in Everyday Life*. New York: Free Press.

Zerubavel, Eviatar. 1996. Lumping and splitting: Notes on social classification. *Sociological Forum* 11 (3):421–33.

Zola, I. K. (1972). Medicine as an institution of social control. *Sociological Review* 20:487–504.

Zola, Irving Kenneth. 1983. *Socio-medical Inquiries: Recollections, Reflections, and Reconsiderations*. Philadelphia: Temple University Press.

Index

Milton Keynes UK
Ingram Content Group UK Ltd.
UKHW010942090624
443798UK00005B/113